PRAISE FOR FLOURISH BEYOND 50

"Flourish Beyond 50: Your Path to Vibrant Living" author Judy Griffin has masterfully combined the wisdom of a host of mind, body and spirit experts and intertwined them with her own personal stories of lessons learned which have resulted in a vibrant life. She spackles the pages with wonderful, nutritional recipes while assuring the reader that the journey is far more simple than many perceive. As you turn the pages you recognize that a cohesive philosophy for harmonious living is unfolding and the reader is left with useful tools and a handy workbook to launch a life of healthy habits and practical principles to living a vibrant life.

— Ariaa Jaeger, Best-Selling author, "Ariaaisms Spiritual Food for the Soul" and "The Book of Ariaa, Quotes for a Luminous Life." www.ariaa.com

"When I first started reading "Flourish", I liked it so much I closed my door and got comfortable, slipping into the comfort and inspiration found on every single page. Judy has a gift for bringing you gently into endless possibility and joy with loving guidance and inspiring self-reflection. Every chapter leads you on a rich journey and she includes fabulous recipes in each chapter that are amazing. For me, this gift of ease should be renamed "Guide to Life" because it has everything I want in one pretty little package. Thank you Judy for the beauty you bring to us all. Christmas shopping just got easier!"

— Carolan Deacon, Healing Songstress, vocalist, speaker, writer and coach www.carolandeacon.com

I was very pleased to read Judy Griffin's book "Flourish Beyond 50". She truly encapsulates the heart of a woman in her writing. We have fears of aging that are needless and she calls us to "Show up!" in all our glory. The design of the book for journaling with insight and the recipes are two of my favorite aspects and were a pleasant surprise among the wisdom and sound recommendations she artfully expresses. This is certainly a book to curl up with and enjoy.

— Dr. Anna Cabeca, Women's Health and Age Management Expert, www.CabecaHealth.com

Flourishing Beyond 50: Your Path to Vibrant Living promotes the continuation of healthy habits and encourages the individual to make lifestyle changes. It is an easy to follow guide that addresses the mind, body and nutrients. The recipes are nutritious and take only a few minutes to prepare. I enjoyed reading this book. As I was reading the stories, I was able to identify several of the characteristics that fit my patients' profiles. That's why I have always taught my patients that being healthy and maintaining health is multi-factorial.

— Dr. Cathleen Gerenger, DC, FIAMA

This is a well written and an inspiring book for anyone who wants to improve their health. So often women don't put themselves first. This books helps you in the comfort of your home do just that. I love all the tools Judy offers, the recipes are great, and the self-reflection exercises are so helpful. Judy says "This book will guide your way" and it certainly does as the chapters are clearly labeled with great ideas and doable actions. This is the type of book to keep next to your bed and refer to when needed. It's a simple read but very powerful and useful.

— Linda Mandelbaum, CHC, theteenhealthcoach.com

I so enjoyed and loved reading every word of this book. So many of us never really allow ourselves to dig deep and consider our true feelings around aging. In "Flourish Beyond 50" Judy comfortably creates a road map that leads her reader from self-discovery to revitalization. With stories, quotes, action steps and recipes this book pleasantly provides a practical, yet soulful guide to "Flourish Beyond 50!"

— Nancy Goggins, CHHC, www.ahealthyfoundation.com

I just finished reading Judy's book and I have to say, if you are over 50, you really need to read this book. I had a touch of "Oh I'm too young to read a book about aging", but once I started to read her chapters, I was immediately drawn into the flow of her voice and wisdom. The book is laid out in a way that each chapter highlights an aspect of a vibrant life and weaves in personal stories of her own and of other women to highlight those points. Each chapter closes with workbook style questions for self-reflection, action steps and a yummy recipe.

I was surprised by how effortlessly the book provided a structure for me to reflect on all of the parts of my life, which I love. Judy succeeded in writing a book that has the voice of sitting down with your best friend and jumping into all those shared experiences and juicy bits that make friendships so valuable. I felt inspired and motivated by each chapter and even psyched to be 50!

Our culture is flooded with books and products on aging, most trying to sell us costly products or magic bullet advice to defy this natural process. The following passage best sums up Judy's awesome grasp on how to truly flourish at any age.

"Although I enjoy select skin care products, supplements, super foods, healing foods, and essential oils that promote vitality, you just can't beat the benefits of play, pleasure, laughter, and love. The truth is simple: your fountain of youth is right inside you. It's in your dreams, your mindset, your attitudes, and your desires. You just need to feed it. Once you rediscover these youthful bene-fits, you'll be ready to embrace them every day."

— Maureen Wheeler, Health Coach & EcoMama
www.itsallconnectedliving.com

Editorial Review

Every so often, I get the rare opportunity to work with an author whose ideas and style mesh so perfectly with my own that I feel like I'm not really working. This is the case with Judy Griffin and her delightfully insightful book, "Flourish Beyond 50: Your Path to Vibrant Living."

Judy and I began working together just weeks before my 48th birthday; needless to say, I am definitely a member of her target audience. What makes her work unique is the honest, graceful manner in which she shares her wisdom (and the insights of women who have touched her life). This is a book about peace, acceptance, joy, appreciation, self-care, and self-love. In so many ways, I feel as though I've been given permission to honor myself, and in so doing, I have moved into a more peaceful and empowering place than ever before.

Within its pages, readers meet a genuine woman whose advice and guidance will make realizing their own dreams simpler than imagined. Judy reminds us to reflect, to move in pleasurable ways, to treat ourselves gently, and to be at home in our own skin. It is an honor to have shared this journey with her, and my copy of her book will be perpetually on my nightstand as a reminder of the gift she has given all women and the power and peace she has given me.

Thank you, Judy. There aren't enough words to express how deeply your words have touched me.

— Tracy Ann Teel, Editor

May you always flourish
in vibrant health.

Judy Griffin

Flourish Beyond 50

YOUR PATH TO VIBRANT LIVING

JUDY GRIFFIN

Cover & Interior by Kayla Griffin
Edited by Tracy Ann Teel

Published by Nourishing Soulutions

Printed in the United States of America

Library of Congress Control Number: 2014918961

ISBN-13:978-0-9908704-0-1

DEDICATION

I dedicate this book to my dad, my brother Joey, my best friend Sue, and all of my friends and family who left us way too soon.

We never know how long we have so it's so important to remember this.

"Each day is a new canvas to paint upon. Make sure your picture is full of life and happiness and at the end of the day you don't look at it and wish you had painted something different."

— Ritu Ghatourey

TABLE OF CONTENTS

ACKNOWLEDGEMENTS

First, I would like to thank my husband for giving me the space to pursue my passion and for always being there for our family. I'm lucky to have married the man of my dreams 25 years ago.

To my wonderful children Kayla, Erin, Conor, and Sean—Being your Mom is my greatest gift and all of you make me proud everyday. You make me laugh, smile, and fill my heart with joy.

I am especially grateful to Kayla for lovingly designing this gorgeous cover and layout with such finesse. I love the beautiful way you have brought my business and book to life.

To my very special Mom who has always been there to love, support, and encourage me. Your understanding, sense of humor, and nurturing mean the world to me.

To my talented sister Lorraine who is always there to lend her support and encouragement. I really value your insight, feedback, and love.

To my stepdad, George— Thank you for stepping into our lives and embracing us with love and kindness.

To my mother and father in law, sister in law, and brother in laws, beautiful nieces and nephews and my very special cousins—I am grateful for your presence in my life.

To Alison Dolan Hall—Thank you for gifting me a yoga class when I needed it most.

To my first yoga teacher, Arlene Lucas—Thank you for guiding my way.

To Kuldip S. Khalsa, my neuromuscular practitioner and yoga teacher. Thank you for helping me to release the sadness and anger so I could heal and embrace the present moment.

To the many lovely yoga teachers I experienced over the last 11 years—Thank you. I am so grateful to have found a home at Divine Yoga and RVC Yoga— a place to flourish.

I am ever so grateful for all of the special family members, friends, teachers, and colleagues who have touched my life. I value our time together.

To Joshua Rosenthal, Founder of Integrative Nutrition—Thank you for encouraging me to embrace a can do attitude. Lindsey Smith— I appreciate the resources and support offered by you and Joshua.

To my supportive editor, Tracy Ann Teel—Your expertise, interest, and guidance have been invaluable.

To my all of my fellow authors, especially Angela Gaffney and Mari Carmen Pizzaro, I really appreciated sharing this journey with you.

Thank you to the women who so graciously contributed their stories to my book. It was an honor to include your meaningful narrative.

Thank you to the many clients I have had the privilege of serving through the years. Our work together has taught me so much and I wrote this book with all of you in mind. The strides you make inspire me every day and you all hold a special place in my heart.

INTRODUCTION

Are you ready to vibrantly embrace a new season in your life?

- One that the calendar doesn't lay out for you?
- One that offers the opportunity to reclaim your zest, essence, and sexy self?
- A season to redefine your purpose, explore your passion, and celebrate your wisdom, sensuality, and grace?
- One to find your best self where you address your needs and desires?
- One where you feed your life, so you can blossom, grow, and thrive?
- One where you cultivate an inner vitality that radiates agelessness?

Every woman, no matter what her circumstance, can make a choice to flourish today. Stepping into the next season is about carving out a life that really suits and serves you. It's finally time to focus on you, your dreams, and desires. Just like a garden, flourishing can look different from one woman to another because we all have unique goals, values, and experiences.

A woman who flourishes shows up in her life and in the life of her friends, family, colleagues, clients, and students. She has confidence, loves herself, has a sense of purpose and passion, is better equipped to voice her feelings and opinions, and, most importantly, she honors, values, and takes care of herself. She feels comfortable in her body and can relax in the present moment. Her inner beauty shows up in her smile, her laugh, and the way she dances through life.

Flourishing is a practice not a destination.

It is a work in progress, and just like yoga, we need to practice flourishing. Of course, we'll experience setbacks along the way, but if our goal is clear, we can always embrace the choices that support our mission.

No Excuses

There is no reason for you to give up on yourself and accept your lack of energy, zest for life, excess weight, health challenges, and hormone havoc as a routine part of aging. Aging is a state of mind, not the active surrender to a withering body and deteriorating mind. Rather, it is a beautiful celebration of this new season of your life where you continue to blossom and feel forever vibrant.

If you seek to avoid succumbing to the pitfalls of aging, then embrace vibrant living by:

- Focusing on your well-being.
- Loving yourself.
- Accepting yourself and owning your choices.
- Venturing away from the aging mindset and embracing youthful vitality.
- Initiating proactive steps to promote longevity.
- Embracing each day with verve, curiosity, and gratitude.
- Finding joy in every day.
- Infusing your life with all those crayons that are still in the box.
- Cultivating a flourishing mindset that kicks aging rhetoric to the curb.

Are you ready to bid farewell to those tired old excuses?

- "Who cares what I wear; no one will be looking at me anyway."
- "That's what happens when you get old."
- "I used to feel beautiful."
- "Who needs sex at our age."
- "I'm too old to wear that."
- "I'd love to … but I'm too old."
- "This disease runs in my family; there's nothing I can do about it."
- "If I were only younger … I'd try it.
- "Well, for a woman of your age … "
- "Is this dress or hair style too young for me?"
- "Just wait until you're my age … you'll see."
- "Declining health, lack of energy, and weight gain are part of aging."

Wouldn't you rather feel Forever Vibrant?

Our attitude, daily choices, and habits shape our lives. Every day we experience challenges, setbacks, and hardships – my life has been no exception. I have learned that even when life deals you a devastating blow, you can still choose well-being. It's in these darkest moments that a lifeline appears, and it's up to us to make sure we grab it.

After I suffered the devastating death of my brother, yoga became my lifeline, and the ripple effect of this choice continues to fuel my flourishing mindset. At 40 years young, that one decision changed everything, and a healthier me emerged. When I found my way back by nourishing the corners of my life, I found a stronger me and began to flourish. This propelled me to seek and cultivate vibrant health, a catalyst in my healing and even in my decision to become a health coach to inspire woman to nourish their way to a vibrant life.

Despite missing my brother's presence, I am so grateful that my 40s were a decade of self-growth, self-awareness, healing, and increased spirituality. This made turning 50 an awesome celebration and prepared me to flourish beyond it. Sadly, like many of us, I know too many women and men who died before reaching their prime, so I view life as a privilege and welcome each passing year because each birthday is a gift that keeps on giving, and we need to cherish it.

My Invitation to You

This book invites you to celebrate your life along with the lives of other women. We can all learn so much from one another. No one has all the answers or a magical secret, but together we can embrace vibrant living. It is essential to listen and learn from the inspiring women you encounter along the way because every women has golden nuggets of wisdom to share. For this reason, I have included real stories from real women who are flourishing and stepping into (or have stepped into) their season of vibrancy.

Meeting, interviewing, and reading their stories has been an enriching and valuable experience. Their experiences add a delightful flavor of inspiration to this book and help guide your way.

This book offers you a path to vibrant living. It's designed to help you navigate your own way and step into this next season with zest, passion, potential, and anticipation. Each chapter celebrates your choice to flourish and opens up another window for vibrant living. You'll find guidance, a nourishing narrative, healthy morsels, meaningful quotes, and inspiration. Look for the Flourish Focus at the end of each chapter that provides a space for self-reflection, to hone in on and explore your thoughts, feelings, dreams, desires, challenges, intentions and well-being. Each Flourish Focus serves up scrumptious recipes and action steps to nourish and support a vibrant lifestyle.

No matter what age you are, you can make the choice to start nourishing your garden today. It's time to embrace your gifts, flourish, and step into your season of vibrancy. This book will guide your way.

CHAPTER 1

Nurturing Your Garden

Nourish To Flourish

When we nourish to flourish
we feel fit, fabulous, vibrant, and beautiful.
Start by nurturing you.
Treat yourself like a garden.
Get rooted in fertile soil that nourishes you.
Plant healthy seeds;
nurture them with plenty of water, sunshine, play, and rest.
Eliminate the weeds that stifle you.
Feed yourself with real food, life food, and soul food
that offer you pleasure, joy, and bliss.
It's not about adhering to a perfect diet or exercise regimen.
It's about discovering what really suits and serves you.
When you embrace the deliciousness of life
and weave in a sense of harmony,
you'll have cultivated a vibrant lifestyle where you thrive
rather than feel deprived or compelled to exercise.

You hear a lot about self-love and self-care, but that wasn't always the case. I remember the first time I was lucky enough to be introduced to these terms. I was watching Oprah while my two baby girls were napping when Dr. Christiane Northrup made her debut. Now, this was a woman that knew how to flourish and was just so at home in her body. I immediately fell in love with her vivacious and captivating presence, so I ordered and embraced every word of **Women's Bodies, Women's Wisdom**. This was the first time I was introduced to the importance of nourishing your body, mind, and soul. Her message encouraging women to embrace and embody self-care and self-love deeply resonated with me.

> *"Caring for yourself is not self-indulgence, it is self-preservation. This is a radical notion for many women who have been taught that self sacrifice is synonymous with being a "good" woman. Have the courage to take care of yourself. That's where world peace begins with you."*

— Dr. Christiane Northrup

Her resourceful books offered me a solid foundation in women's wellness. 20 years later, they remain my go-to guides. It was then that I decided I would strive to be a well-nourished woman who flourishes.

How to Begin

Flourishing starts with you, and the more you nourish, the more you'll flourish. All too often, women focus their attention on others while omitting themselves from the equation. As parents, nurturers, caretakers, and practitioners, we can easily get lost in the shuffle. It's vital to remember that when we self-nourish, we thrive, which enables us to nurture our loved ones more fully. Remember that self-care isn't an indulgence but is vital to your well-being and that of your family's and the people you serve.

Even when we are experiencing challenging times, it is so important to remember that we have a choice in every circumstance, so look for something positive and embrace it. In order to step into your season of vibrancy, it's essential that you realize there is plenty of time for you to blossom and grow.

You can blossom like a luscious garden with:
- Sleep and rest
- Water and nutritious foods
- Support
- Friendship/Companionship
- Peace/Silence/Meditation
- Flow-fitness, stretching, and movement
- Pleasure and fun
- Love
- Faith/Spirituality
- Joy
- Gratitude

Consider the healthy seeds you can plant:
- Joy
- Faith
- Goals
- Hobbies/Activities
- Forgiveness/Acceptance

- Positivity
- Compassion
- Connection/Relationships/Friendships
- Motivation
- Determination/Passion/Purpose

Be mindful of the weeds that keep you from flourishing:

- Stress
- Toxins
- Negativity
- Unhealthy relationships
- Baggage
- Junk
- Unhappy careers
- Illness
- Unhealthy habits

My Journey

There was a point in my life when my health and well-being was compromised, and I discovered that one decision changed everything, and a healthier me emerged. After the tragic loss of my brother, I really lost myself in sadness. My overwhelming grief led to an unhealthy habit that took a toll on me and my whole family. Now, I'm all for enjoying some cocktails, but I was using wine to lull myself to sleep, and this just wasn't serving me since the lulling effects would wear off and nightmares would wake me up. I just wasn't showing up in my life.

I was also experiencing extreme facial pain, which I assumed was a sinus infection. To my surprise, after a clear MRI scan, the neurologist prescribed a mild sedative to relieve the neuralgia-like symptoms brought on by mild depression. The very next day I was scheduled to attend an introductory yoga class and luncheon given by my lovely friend, Alison. Even though I had never practiced yoga, somehow my soul knew it would help, and I am so glad I listened. In that moment, I knew if I started taking the sedative I would never know if the yoga worked. Would it be the sedative or the yoga?

Choosing Yoga

I started yoga the next day without ever filling that prescription. Yoga became my lifeline and guided me to a healthier me. Consistently practicing yoga lit up every corner of my life and continues to light my way. I started sleeping like a baby and no longer needed to use wine to soothe my soul. Not to say I don't enjoy a glass of wine or two.

What I discovered was how much I needed stillness because busy was always easy for me and stillness was a challenge. At first, the most difficult pose was Savasana, which is the final essential relaxation pose used to rest that gives your body time to integrate the experience. I used to think about leaving class early to avoid this pose of stillness, which required me to lay motionless for 10 minutes, but I stuck with it, and it became a cherished pose that I now fully embrace. Early on, I often struggled to keep up, and my teacher said, "I'll know you're doing yoga when you let your breath guide you, and I see you surrender in child's pose and rest."

The day I stopped pushing and surrendered to my breath was groundbreaking because I learned to live my yoga practice off the mat and listen to myself in ways that I never had before. This propelled me to seek and cultivate vibrant health by focusing on self-nourishment and self-care while cultivating a voracious appetite for holistic modalities that promoted well-being.

Eating for Wellness

On my quest to thrive, I experienced my first cleanse, and it changed my relationship with food. I learned how foods heal, energize, and impact your mood and well-being. Eating delicious and nutritious foods is also another way to love myself. From that cleanse, I honed in on foods that truly nourished me and discovered those that compromised my health. Harnessing the healing power of food helped me zero in on my passion for wellness, and led me to enroll in the Professional Health Coach Training Program at Integrative Nutrition. This cleanse made such a vital impact on my health that it remains a cornerstone of my health coaching practice. Eating for wellness is a gift rather than a deprivation, and I am passionate about sharing this with you.

https://nourishingsoulutions.com/work-with-me/fall-cleanse/

Flourish Focus

"When you recover or discover something that nourishes your soul and brings joy, care enough about yourself to make room for it in your life."

– Jean Bolen

Self-Reflection:
What will help your garden blossom?

_____

_____

_____

_____

_____

What healthy seeds can you plant?

_____

_____

_____

_____

_____

What weeds are keeping you from flourishing?

_____

_____

_____

_____

_____

Life can be so tasty when you discover what makes it delicious.
How can you embrace the deliciousness in your life?

_____

_____

_____

_____

_____

Action Step: Carve out time every day to nourish your garden in some way.

Here are five simple ways to nourish your garden:

1. Start your day with a nourishing breath series.
2. Nourish, cleanse, and hydrate your body with a daily cup of warm water with ½ of a freshly squeezed lemon. Drink eight glasses of water throughout the day.
3. Engage in daily fitness activities that make your body feel good.
4. Nourish yourself with nutrient dense delicious foods that pleasure your palate.
5. Connect with a family member, friend, or lover every day.

Nourishing Breath Series:

This will help avoid the shallow breathing that most of us engage in.

1. Lay down on back with both hands on your belly.
2. Inhale deeply for five seconds.
3. Notice your belly inflating. Breathe deeply from your belly in this pose and in life.
4. Exhale deeply for five seconds and notice your belly deflating.
5. Repeat five times.

Recipe: Roasted Butternut Rainbow Salad

When you eat vibrantly, you feel more vibrant.

Serves 4-6

Ingredients:

- 1 small butternut squash – about 2 lbs.
- 4 cups baby spinach – about 8 oz.
- 2 Tbsp extra-virgin coconut oil
- 1 tsp ground turmeric
- 1 tsp minced fresh ginger
- 1 tsp cinnamon
- 1 tsp Celtic Sea Salt
- ¼ red onion, finely chopped
- ¼ cup dried cranberries
- ¼ cup crushed pecans
- seeds of 1 pomegranate

Dressing:

- 1 cup (lightly packed) roughly chopped fresh basil leaves
- 1 garlic clove, peeled and finely minced
- ¼ cup extra-virgin olive oil
- ¼ cup nutritional yeast
- 2 Tbsp raw apple cider vinegar (I like Bragg's best)
- 1 Tbsp raw honey
- 1 lemon, freshly squeezed

Cook quinoa while squash is roasting.

1. Rinse 1 cup of quinoa
2. Add to 2 cups of water in a pot and bring to boil.
3. Lower heat and simmer about 10–15 minutes, until water is absorbed.

Directions:

1. Preheat oven to 400.
2. Prick squash with a fork and roast until slightly tender, about 15 minutes.
3. Remove squash from oven, cut open, and scoop out seeds (*save seeds to roast later*).
4. Cut squash into cubes (*It's easier to cube once it has roasted a bit*).
5. Toss the squash with turmeric, minced fresh ginger, cinnamon, sea salt, and coconut oil.
6. Roast until lightly browned and tender, about 15 minutes.

Prepare dressing while squash is roasting:

1. Combine basil, garlic, and nutritional yeast in a blender until smooth.
2. Add olive oil and vinegar. Process until smooth. Set aside.

Salad:

1. Mix roasted squash, spinach, pomegranate seeds, onions, pecans, and cranberries in bowl.
2. Thoroughly mix in dressing.
3. Serve over quinoa and enjoy. Serve warm or cold.

See more at https://www.nourishingsoulutions.com/roasted-butternut-rainbow-salad

Guiding Words from Flourish Contributor, Polly Leaf

I met Polly Leaf in yoga class and have always admired her beauty, grace, vibrancy, flexibility, and youthful attitude. Polly was a gifted kindergarten teacher and also a gardener at heart. She nurtures her own gardens just as beautifully as she nourishes herself. I admire Polly's honesty, the vivacious way she embraces life, and the fine example she sets for flourishing at any age.

—

I am 75 and chronology doesn't mean much to me. I don't know what feeling "old" means. I embrace every single moment of every single day.

There have been times when I had to choose between sticking with the old ways or stepping into the unknown. I have focused on the more adventuresome route, the one that opened me up to more beauty, joy, and opportunities.

For way too long, I was hypercritical of just about every-thing, including other people. Unable to take action because of this attitude, it finally dawned on me that the person I was most critical of was myself. Over time, I have recognized that I have more to offer than I ever thought. I now step into new ventures with joy and gratitude, and I have become less critical of myself and of others.

Along the way I learned that my own negative thinking prevented me from accomplishing things, maintaining relationships, and from just about everything. When I believe in myself, I can do anything.

It has taken me many years, too many, to understand that the most important thing is to love myself, and that once that begins, life becomes a positive, treasured experience.

Back in the 80s, I decided to live more vibrantly after reading, Out On a Limb, by Shirley MacLaine. In the book, she mentioned a retreat at an ashram in California that was extremely rigorous and consisted mostly of hiking and yoga. I decided to follow her advice and experienced five transformative days and was able to complete an 18 mile hike in the San Gabriel mountains by the end of my stay. I felt totally renewed.

I left committed to fitness and to facing challenges with a "can do" attitude. I returned three more times and know that exercise is key to my physical, emotional, and spiritual well being, and at this point in time, yoga suits me best.

Taking care of myself first is truly the best way to serve others. Meditation and yoga nourish my soul. I nurture myself by eating and preparing organic wholesome meals, spending time with family and friends, reading, painting, sketching, gardening, traveling, playing with my dog, and listening to music.

With the gift of wisdom, I would tell the younger me to trust my intuition and to think more independently, rather than follow others. I would not be as concerned about other people's opinions. I would believe in myself.

CHAPTER 2

Designing Each Decade

"*If it's true your life flashes past your eyes before you die, then it is also the truth that your life rushes forth when you are ready to start to truly be alive.*"

— Amy Hempel, The Collected Stories

Designing Each Decade

What phase of life are you living right now? You may be happily married, happily single, widowed, or divorced. As we approach our 50s, our lives are often in flux based on the paths we took. Many are getting accustomed to an empty nest while others have half in the nest and half out, and some have a long way to go, and still others never had a nest. There are women enjoying life-long fulfilling careers while others are seeking to retire. And many women are ready to pursue their passions and discover or redefine their purposes.

Whatever stage you are in, it's key to prepare for the shifts your life will take in order to avoid stagnating. Perhaps you have already experienced shifts that you have yet to address. This is a perfect perch from which to view your life and define how the next season will look.

Coping with Tragedy

It is impossible to journey through life unscathed by disease, misfortune, unforeseen circumstance, or tragedy. To varying degrees, by the time we reach our 50s, most of us have experienced some type of game changer. My heart goes out to all of you who have suffered or are still trying to overcome from a serious health issue, painful loss, setback, or negative experience. There are certain things we never get over but rather learn to live with instead.

It's vital for me to point out that there are no easy answers when it comes to picking up the pieces after the unexpected happens. The area I live in was deeply affected by the tragedies of September 11th. Families in Rockville Centre, NY and neighboring towns experienced unfathomable loss. My little children and I were very lucky that my husband came home that day since he worked at the World Trade Center. Tragically, many 30 and 40 something wives, teens, children, and toddlers lost their loved ones that day. My heart continues to go out to these families, and they serve as a continual reminder for me to cherish each day.

You don't have to go far to meet someone who suffered from that day. Just yesterday I ran into a lovely women on the beach that offered to take a picture of my husband and me with our sons. She said that they reminded her of her boys at that age and then shared that they all enjoyed surfing with her husband— another good man taken that day.

Sadly, I've also known many women who have lost their husbands early to heart attacks, cancer, and other diseases. There are also women facing divorce as they enter this next season. So, what do you do when life takes away the future you had planned? Unfortunately, there are no easy answers here. All I can say is take it moment by moment, get plenty of support, feel your feelings, be with people you love, deeply nourish yourself, and soothe your soul. I am always struck by the resiliency I witness in women who have been forced to carve out "a new normal" and redesign a life they hadn't expected.

Own Your Choices

At this pivotal time in your life, your daily choices matter because they set the tone for decades to come. You have the opportunity to change the course of your life, so choose the life you want to lead and plan for it. If you want to feel fit, fabulous, and vibrant, then it's essential to carve out a healthy lifestyle at once.

All too often we hear about the negative aspects of aging, and we can easily fall into the trap of assuming that they define aging. Weight gain and low energy, being out of shape, having a lackluster life or low libido, chronic health issues and disease, and conversations about hip or knee replacement seem synonymous with growing older. Although this may be true for some women, remember, you choose the life you want to live. Do you plan on flourishing with ageless vibrancy or watching the days pass by uneventfully?

It's up to us to decide if we want to be the 80-year-old woman dancing at the party or the one confined to a wheel chair. Of course, we can't prevent every ailment— weak joints or disease— but we can certainly strive to steer our lives in a healthy and fulfilling direction. No one wants to be a young woman trapped in an old body, so make the effort to thrive.

Get to the Heart of Your Ailments

I really feel for women who suddenly find themselves in an aging body. You can feel strong and healthy one day, and suddenly that can be taken away. Even if you are suffering from a chronic disease or health issue, now is the time to make sure your medical team has uncovered the root cause of your condition because the band-aid approach won't serve you well or promote longevity. It is important to avoid attributing your symptoms to aging or hormone imbalances, like I did, because sometimes there is an illness or condition that needs to be diagnosed. Last year I blamed my excessive fatigue on my hormones only to find out a few months later that I had mono.

Your lifestyle most certainly impacts your life. When you nurture yourself, you take charge of your health. So why not make the choices that offer you a vivacious, zest filled life? As a health coach, my goal is to help women nourish their way to vibrant lives. You

can learn more here: https://www.nourishingsoulu-
tions.com

Show Up in Your Life

Along with some wrinkles, we can take measures
to be healthy and fit with a youthful mindset.
It starts by showing up in our lives and making
proactive decisions that keep us strong, energized,
and engaged. Envision yourself growing into your
future with vitality, adventure, vibrancy, grace,
fulfillment, joy, and beauty. This requires a dedica-
tion to your well-being, a plan, and a mindset that
supports your goals.

> *"Today is my tomorrow. It's up to me to shape it, to
> take control and seize every opportunity. The power is
> in the choices I make each day. I eat well.
> I live well. I shape me."*

— Anonymous

You Can Always Set a New Course

At any given point you can redirect the compass of
your life, set your sight on the woman you want to
be, and navigate the life you want to live. Consider
how you are showing up in your life. Because no
matter your age, you can take an inventory of where
you are at and consider where you want to be and
then go for it.

For instance, if your goal is to cut your risk of disease
and maintain an optimal weight range, then that's
going to require a lifestyle that favors nutritious

foods, adequate rest, stress management, and physical activity. You can't spend your time watching TV, indulging in chips, soda, or wine, and expect to thrive in the next decade.

The Surprising Cumulative Effect

The choices we make in each decade accumulate, and the impact of unhealthy choices magnifies with each new decade. We got away with a lot in our teens and 20s, but as we mature our choices catch up with us. Ever notice how your body can't tolerate junk food, alcohol, soda, or caffeine like it did when you were younger? What about when you take a break from your fitness routine and feel out of shape when you return to it? You wont wake up and magically become someone you're not, but whatever decade you are in, you can choose to live vibrantly and turn your life around.

Over time, we grow accustomed to our habits and choices, which make it more challenging to veer in new directions. This is why the lifestyle you practice in each decade so greatly impacts the next one. So, strive to cultivate a healthier lifestyle today that offers you a fruitful future. Otherwise, you can be a 60-year-old living in a 90-year-old woman's body if you don't reign yourself in. I think we would all rather feel forever young.

Embrace Your True Desires

"You are never too old to set another goal or to dream a new dream."

— C. S. Lewis

As you notice that your role is shifting as the landscape of your life takes on a new shape, it's vital to consider how you want to feel and what you want to do as you embrace the next season. This is how we can design each decade to live a life that uniquely suits us. When you prioritize your dreams and ambitions, you can attain the life you envision if you make a plan and take the action steps to get to your destination.

For instance, if you've been waiting all your life to travel, then take preventative measures to avoid hobbling around Europe. If you run yourself ragged in your 40s, 50s, and 60s, you may not be healthy enough to reap the rewards of retirement or an adventurous lifestyle. Even if early retirement isn't feasible, you can create a career or business that affords you income and flexibility.

If you have a fulfilling career you enjoy, postponing retirement may serve you best. Sometimes when women retire prematurely and are unsure of their plans for the next season, their lives may feel very unfulfilling. Often, when children leave the nest, women feel out of sorts since their kids were always their primary focus. Conversely, other women may just be tickled pink because they have time to read, relax, hit the beach, socialize with friends, or embrace community service.

Keep in mind that it isn't always essential to know the specifics as long as you have an idea of how you want your life to feel. This idea can guide your way, and flexibility is key when navigating through your life and planning for the next decade. We can't possibly know what is coming our way, so it is necessary to cultivate a mindset that can go with the flow just a bit. Illness, loss, tragedies, family issues, and job changes can easily change the course of the life we imagined and require us to navigate our way in uncharted waters.

I know all too well how major losses can turn your life upside down. It certainly isn't easy acclimating to unforeseen circumstances and a life never imagined. Even so, a choice must be made that allows us to find our way back to ourselves and to a new normal. Certainly, a supple, buoyant, and resilient nature will help women endure the curveballs and weather the storms that turn up in their lives.

Flourish Focus

"The way you think, the way you behave, the way you eat, can influence your life by 30 to 50 years."

— Deepak Chopra

Self-Reflection:

When have you felt like your life was in sync? What made you feel that way?

_____

_____

_____

_____

_____

_____

_____

_____

How could you harness the qualities of this time and use it today?

_____

_____

_____

_____

How do you feel about aging? What are your expectations?

_____

_____

_____

_____

What kind of life are you designing? How do you want to live? Does this complement the lifestyle you designed?

_____

_____

_____

_____

Action Steps:

1. Initiate three action steps this week to improve the quality of your life and health. Keep it super simple – i.e. drink more water, eat a healthy breakfast, take a yoga class, go for a walk, cook a nourishing meal.

_____

_____

_____

2. Start writing down your dreams and desires in a journal.

Recipe: Sunny Yellow Split Pea Soup

Cook up some sunshine.

Makes 4 ample servings

Ingredients:

- 2 cups dried yellow split peas
- 8 cloves of garlic
- 1 large onion, chopped
- 2 tsp Celtic Sea Salt
- 6 cups water
- ¼ cup fresh lemon juice (*optional*)
- 2 Tbsp chopped fresh dill (*or 2 tsp dried dill*)
- Freshly ground black pepper to taste
- Sprinkle with paprika (*optional*)
- 1 sprig of fresh dill (*optional*)

Directions:

1. Rinse peas and combine with garlic cloves, onion, salt, and water in a large pot.
2. Bring to a boil, cover, and simmer for 30 minutes.
3. Blend soup in the pot with a handheld blender until smooth.
4. Add lemon juice, dill, and paprika, and season with pepper to taste and serve.

See more at https://nourishingsoulutions.com/sunny-yellow-split-pea-soup

Guiding Words from Flourish Contributor, Jane Stinson

Jane is a strong and determined woman, licensed massage therapist, and Certified Health Coach, who I had the privilege of mentoring while she was enrolled at the Institute for Integrative Nutrition.

—

The summer after my sophomore year in high school was a time in my life when I felt self-confident, powerful, happy, content, and comfortable in my own skin. I felt confident in my decision to choose a college track. I was 15, fit, cute, working 40 hours per week, making great money, and feeling wonderful and comfortable in my own skin.

My mom, a cautious woman, encouraged me to acquire secretarial skills since we couldn't afford college, and said this was the sensible route and would make me more marketable. By the end of the summer, the "good girl" Jane, who always did what she was told, caved. The next year I started dating my husband, got engaged at 18, married at 20, and never went to college.

All of us can remember a time when we felt strong, even if for only a moment. A time when we owned our own power and knew what we wanted, where we were going, and were moving and grooving in life.

So, here I am. I raised two children successfully, went through a divorce, recreated myself, and am building my business. I do not want to be 15 again, but I do want to connect with that energy of self-worth, determination, and the pearl in the oyster.

I am not suggesting that I do not have moments, hours, or days of owning who I am, but during that 15th summer, I had a consistent feeling of strength and could not be knocked down by the actions of others.

Here's the deal: it is never too late to start over. Even if you never felt like the world was your oyster, you can, step by step, create practices to make your goals and dreams a reality. I am very clear about who I am and am dedicated to learning lessons and creating joy in my life and the life of my clients and family.

At every age we can recreate ourselves, play big, be in action, and never be defined by what others think or say about us! Take a deep breath, dream a dream, mourn the past but don't live there, and get the show on the road.

CHAPTER 3

Embracing Your Wisdom, Grace, & Sensuality

With each passing year, we gain self-awareness and become more comfortable with our place in life. Our vast experiences help us to evolve into wise, self-assured women comfortable in our own shoes. One of the best things about getting older is that we appreciate our gifts, accept our weaknesses, and love ourselves for who we are. In fact, what we once deemed to be a weakness might have actually been a strength in disguise.

The Gift of Wisdom

Each decade offers a much more vivid vantage point. Wisdom is one of the greatest perks of aging. Just think about how much wiser and more sensible you are now than you were at 18, 25, 30, and 40.

Just think of all of the misguided assumptions you made as a young woman. The learning curve of life really starts paying valuable dividends with each passing year. Of course, now we could redo certain moments in our lives with finesse, but there is no need to focus on past mistakes since they offered valuable lessons. The best use of a woman's wisdom is to carve out a flourishing future.

What Was the Younger You Like?

Mine was indecisive. She lacked confidence, didn't always believe in herself, wasn't very assertive, and wanted everyone to get along. Once a young girl afraid of her own shadow, I really appreciate the self-assurance I developed over time. The younger me didn't know what self-care or self-love was. She was a people pleaser and wanted everyone to like her. Like you, her journey was just beginning. With each passing year, she grew wiser thanks to life's ups and downs. She learned from her experiences and from other women. And she discovered something very important about us all— once we fully accept ourselves, we blossom.

I have found that confidence grows when you override self-doubt, feel the fear, and do it any way. Fear of being wrong used to prevent me from volunteering an answer, but now I readily offer my opinion. Self-assurance emerges with wisdom, and as self-doubt dissipates confidence swells. It's learning that what makes us unique is a strength to be cherished. It's like discovering your very own free square. Since many young women lack confidence, this is a most welcome gift. It certainly was for me.

"In life, we each have a free square. Something that comes naturally or easily to us but not to others. We may not think too much about it or disregard it altogether. Once you identify your free squares, play them by using what's easy to help you with what isn't."

— Victoria Moran, Creating a Charmed Life

Breaking from Conformity

As young women, we are often indecisive, and fear prevents us from voicing our desires. Our younger selves found it easier to conform rather than stand out. We stifled our feelings to avoid hurting others. This was true for me. As a young woman, I was uncomfortable standing up for myself. I always felt more comfortable as the peacemaker, the one who got along with everyone, but somewhere along the way I realized this behavior can compromise your health. It is so important for women to voice their opinions, concerns, beliefs, discontent, desires, and dreams. As a young woman, I couldn't voice my feelings without becoming emotional. This gradually evolved as my confidence began emerging in my late 20s. Thankfully, I no longer break into tears when I'm engaged in heated discussions. This is a huge step in growing from a girl to a woman and is a skill to be admired in young women. It's vital to veer away from being a people pleaser and to concentrate on pleasing yourself first. A truly confident woman believes in herself, isn't focused on her likeability factor, offers a warm smile, and shows up as herself.

"I do not accept my age — I celebrate it! I wear my wrinkles, silver hair, and age spots as medals of honor. Life and beauty is all what you make it. That is what attractiveness and aging gracefully is all about. Enjoy it!"

— Cindy Joseph

The Gift of Grace

As women blossom, the sands of time offer the gift of grace. Grace comes in many forms. It isn't necessarily defined as an impeccably dressed, tall, gorgeous woman with perfect posture. Grace accepts who she is, shows up as herself, offers ease, and doesn't worry since that interferes with enjoying the present moment. She is light-hearted, kind, welcoming, and has blossomed joyfully over time. And the beauty of this gift is that anyone can connect to the goddess within and garner the grace she exudes since grace rises with self-nourishment, love, and acceptance. She has a beautiful presence, smiles and laughs with ease, and doesn't rush since she always has time. A graceful woman loves herself and doesn't wear her age, although she accepts it. Meryl Streep wears grace well. I appreciate her words,

"You have to embrace getting older. Life is precious, and when you've lost a lot of people you realize that each day is a gift."

Connecting to Our Sensual Essence

With the wisdom, confidence, and grace we've garnered, we can open one of the best gifts of growing into ourselves – the connection to our essence – which was waiting for us all along. This is where we meet sensuality.

Do you feel comfortable embracing your sensuality? Many women don't because of the sexual connotation, but sensuality encompasses so much more than that. It means tuning into your senses and finding pleasure in the food you eat and the places you visit, the clothes you wear and the way you feel. Enjoying the music you hear, the people you touch, the activities you enjoy, and the choices you make are all part of your sensual nature. Although we desire intimacy and companionship, it is not a prerequisite for feeling sensual. Sensuality immerses you in the present moment and lights up your awareness.

Sensuality embraces life, knows what makes her feel good, and is comfortable in her own skin. She loves herself up, likes to feel loved, and be in love. A sensual woman appreciates her body without focusing on her "flaws." In fact, she may be ready to look past her "flaws" and to step out of the darkness. Sensuality can be accessed anywhere – in a chocolate delight, among the ticklish blades of soft grass, or in the softly setting sun on a beach. Whatever your pleasure, perhaps diving into a wave, breathing in the ocean air or a luscious garden, enjoying your lover's embrace, or simply wearing your favorite dress, sensuality is everywhere. It is a welcome blessing refined over time. Sophia Loren epitomizes sensuality, but it comes in all shapes and forms and rises from within.

Honor Yourself

It's important to note that when we have too much on our plate, find ourselves rushing from place to place, and aren't prioritizing self-care, we aren't able to embrace grace, wisdom, and sensuality. I know this to be true and find that my sensuality rises when I honor myself with rejuvenating activities, silence, and space. Running by the ocean, practicing yoga, swimming, deep breathing, and meditation awakens me, connects me to my essence, and turns on my sensuality.

If you are looking to get your sexy back, feeling more sensual is key. I'm not talking about what you see in magazines but rather the sexy inside you. It's about feeling sexy and beautiful simply for you. It starts in your brain and flows throughout your body.

Refresh and Relax

Time really shrinks when we are stressed, but when we engage in replenishing activities, time expands. I learned this important lesson by attending a mini yoga retreat that I didn't think I had time for because I had to prepare for my son's communion party. I waffled about going but reaped so many benefits as a result. Because I had the chance to relax my mind, my calmness washed over the entire family since no one was put in the position of reacting to a haggard mom trying to get it all done. I ran some errands that morning and every light was green and every line moved quickly. I'm certain that time expanded that day, and I always try to focus on this lesson when I am feeling crazed.

Flourish Focus

"It is confidence in our bodies, minds, and spirits that allows us to keep looking for new adventures, new directions to grow in, and new lessons to learn – which is what life is all about."

— Marlene Dietrich

Self-Reflection:

What would the wiser you tell your younger you?

_____

_____

_____

_____

When did you feel your confidence emerging?

_____

_____

_____

_____

How does grace appear in your life?

_____

_____

_____

_____

What makes you feel sensual?

_____

_____

_____

_____

What's your Free Square?

_____

_____

_____

_____

Action Steps:

- Nurture your sensuality with relaxation and rejuvenation.
- Get a massage or roll a tennis ball under your feet for a relaxing foot massage.
- Buy or wear lingerie or an outfit that makes you feel sexy and special.
- Make a date with yourself or a loved one.
- Luxuriate in a relaxing candle lit bath.

  Stress Relieving Soothing Bath Recipe
  - 2 cups Epsom salt
  - ½ cup baking soda
  - 10 drops lavender oil

Recipe: Roasted Chickpeas with Chopped Spinach

Deep nourishment feeds our sensuality.

Serves 4-6

Ingredients:

- 1 16 oz. can of organic chickpeas (*I prefer the brand Eden*)
- 1 cup halved organic grape tomatoes
- 2 cloves garlic, chopped
- 1 Tbsp of olive oil
- 1 Tbsp parsley
- 2 Tbsp oregano (*dried or fresh*)
- Celtic Sea Salt to taste
- 2 cups of chopped spinach (*Swiss chard & kale can also be used*)

Directions:

1. Drain and rinse chickpeas
2. Mix chickpeas with all ingredients except spinach.
3. Roast in oven at 400 degrees for about 30-40 minutes (*depending on your preferred level of crispiness*)
4. In the last 10 minutes mix in chopped spinach.
5. Cook 10 additional minutes and serve.

See more at: https://nourishingsoulutions.com/chick-pea-stuffed-endive/

Guiding Words from Flourish Contributor, Carolan Deacon

Although I've never met Carolan in person, I feel like I have since her beautiful words, voice, and encouragement have nourished and soothed me ever since I met her in an online forum. Carolan is like a gracious fairy, sharing her enchanted voice and loving heart, and sprinkles ease and grace wherever she goes.

—

I feel more alive now, at the age of 43, than I ever have in my life.

I enjoy better health now, at the age of 43, than I ever have in my life.

I am happier now, at the age of 43, than I ever have been in my life.

I am flourishing now, at the age of 43...and I am grateful.

My journey is not so special, but what I learned along the way I am happy to share with you along with my loving intention that it lifts, inspires, and guides you to your next step toward flourishing...at any age.

I struggled from a young age with anxiety, low self-esteem, and no healthy sense of who I was and what would fulfill me. I grasped at a lot of mistruths and false substances to 'help' me. And down I went.

Fast-forward 10 years to 2002. I decided at 32 that I wanted to let go of my crutches and live the life I knew was waiting for me. I made some huge lifestyle changes, which included a divorce, a total health makeover, and a career change. I also embraced my God with all my heart. I wrapped myself in Spirit like a warm blanket. I changed my life 360 degrees.

Was it quick? No. Was it easy? Yes ... once I let go of my resistance to letting go and letting God. It was easy when I learned to trust my intuition. And it is this that I want to emphasize to you — I had an inner compass. I knew it when I made bad choices. I knew it when I veered off the path to my highest good. I knew it when I listened to Spirit and said 'yes.'

Listen, dear one, listen to your heart's whisper. It is God and will never lead you astray. Three years ago, I had a heart whisper to create a music ministry to help others live vibrantly, sharing my own positive music with imagery, sound, and affirmative lyrics in a way that serves. I am now traveling all over the country sharing my gifts of music.

One and a half years ago, I had a heart whisper to create an online program and community supporting women to cope with stress and life changes naturally. I created Ease and Grace and now guide amazing women from all over the world.

Three and a half years ago, I listened to my intuition and sought help from a reflexologist. I then had the deepest heart whisper come true as my daughter was born. She is the greatest gift and the beat of my heart. She landed in my arms with the smile of God on her face. And I am so grateful...so blessed.

CHAPTER 4

Nourishing You

Our attitude, daily choices, and habits shape our lives. If it's your choice to live vivaciously and thrive, nourishing your body, mind, heart, and soul is vital. Consuming a daily dose of real food, life food, and soul food breathes freshness into your life, so you can live vibrantly. Neglecting this vital sustenance consistently can compromise your health, but your life can blossom like a luscious garden if you feed it well.

Real Food consists of the daily meals, drinks, snacks, and desserts you consume. The quality of the food you eat impacts your health, so it's important to evaluate how home cooked meals, take-out meals, fast food, junk food, and fresh and wholesome foods fit into your daily routine. Your eating habits make an impact on how well real food nourishes you, but how, what, and with whom you eat also counts. No matter how nutritious your diet is, you need to nourish yourself beyond food to live vibrantly.

Life Food includes the joyful, fulfilling, relaxing, and nourishing activities you engage in that connect you to your family, friends, purpose, livelihood, community, and yourself. Flourish by feeling satiated in these facets of life food: family, friendship, fulfillment, fitness, and fun. When you think about what's on your plate every day, you realize that your hobbies, leisure and work activities, responsibilities, relationships, private time, and intimacy are all on the menu. It's what we need to feel vivacious, energized, stimulated, and radiant. It keeps us in the game of life and offers us a vital form of nourishment. Life food lights up your life and ignites your passion for living.

Soul Food is more than just a type of cuisine. For women, soul food is a way of connecting to our essence, spirituality, faith, higher purpose, and ourselves. Silence and stillness are key when accessing our inner compass, which helps guide our way. Focusing on self-love and self-care, exploring your role in life, and delving into personal growth will deepen this connection. Nurturing your soul with joyful acts, meditation, breathing exercises, yoga, praying, and worship creates a healing oasis within. Exploring ways to soothe yourself is pure nourishment for the soul. (Download a soul soother's guide at https://nourishingsoulutions.com/free-gift/)

When I was enrolled at the Institute for Integrative Nutrition, Joshua Rosenthal, the school's founder, introduced these terms as Primary Food and Secondary Food.

"The more I observed human behavior, the more convinced I became that the key to health is understanding each person's individual needs rather than following a set of predetermined rules. I saw plenty of evidence that having happy relationships, a fulfilling career, an exercise routine, and a spiritual practice are even more important to health than a daily diet."

— Joshua Rosenthal

Choose to Flourish

Treating food as the fuel that makes your body run will motivate you to make savvier and healthier choices. The more vibrant and colorful your food is the more revitalized you will feel. These choices increase your energy and affinity to engage in joyous activities that help you to feel fit and fabulous and to flourish.

How's Your Mood?

We don't always realize that our choices are weighing us down in more ways than one, both mentally and physically. Picture a highly processed colorless meal verses a colorful rainbow of nutritious flavorful food. The first will likely increase fatigue, stress, and even promote a bad mood, while the latter choice will make us feel energized and healthy. If you're feeling depressed, nervous, jittery, heavy, restless, hostile, and impatient, it may be related to the food choices you have made. Wholesome choices can make us feel happier, sexier, friendlier, lighter, and healthier, and they also increase clarity, creativity, and ambition. Choices feed off themselves, so you can easily spiral downward by continuing to make choices that don't serve you. This is especially true as we cross into the next season. As we approach our 50s, our bodies have less tolerance for alcohol, sugar, and refined foods. Remember how easy it was to bounce back in your 20s? Unhealthy choices just didn't catch up to us as quickly. The great news is that consistent healthy choices can quickly accumulate and cultivate the vibrancy you're seeking. This is the ripple effect you've been searching for.

> *"Eating well becomes another way that we demonstrate self-love, a greater connection to our soul."*

— Maureen Whitehouse

Assess Your Choices

When we fuel our bodies, we nourish ourselves from within, and we can show up in the world with energy, passion, lightness, and purpose. The more vibrant the food, the more vibrant you will feel, act, and look. Nutritious and delicious meals pleasure our palate and tell us from our cells to our souls that we matter. Ever notice how well nourished you feel when you eat a scrumptious meal prepared with love and care?

It is also important to assess your level of nourishment, especially when you feel out of sorts, because lapses in soul, life, or real food can impact you in a number of ways. When women are lacking in life or soul food, they can easily succumb to excessive behavior like using food to soothe their needs, alleviate stress, and suppress anger. This turns into a vicious cycle because their needs can't be satiated with food. Loneliness often leads to indulging in choices that don't serve our vitality. Some clients have shared their unwillingness to cook for one, so they end up eating junk just because they lack self-worth. A bowl of ice cream or a bag of chips can easily become a woman's best friend when she feels isolated. To avoid this behavior, I encourage you to cook up delicious meals that can be repurposed for additional meals, invite friends over to eat, join a cooking club, and remind yourself that you are worth it. Taking time to check in and nourish yourself fully will help you to flourish by feeding your body, mind, and soul.

The Benefit of Choosing You

Ageless vibrancy doesn't just happen over night but rather is cultivated over time. It requires commitment. Taking care of everyone else while sacrificing your own care is a trap women easily fall into. It's essential to choose you because when you do your loved ones will reap the benefits.

"Self-nurturing is far more than pampering; it is about returning home to your heart."

— Jennifer Loudon

What Are You Really Hungry For?

Your mindset really matters and plays a crucial role in driving your choices. Increased awareness helps establish a healthy mindset and helps you learn what you are really hungry for. It's just not as simple as following a specific diet of do's and don'ts. How many times do you grab a pretzel, a cookie, or a candy bar because you are really just bored, tired, stressed, unfulfilled, or frustrated? This is a clear signal that food is being used to fill a void, and you should consider the feelings behind the cravings.

Vibrant health isn't just about eating an abundance of greens and adhering to a fitness regimen. When you are stressed out, frustrated, weary, and disenchanted, "an ideal diet" and exercise can only take you so far. It's essential to find your essence and develop a sense of balance that makes you feel completely at home in your body, in your actions, and in your life.

The Stress Factor

Women often increase stress by holding on to grudges, trying to be perfect, being too hard on and expecting too much from themselves, and disregarding their own needs. It's no secret that stress compromises our health and interferes with our nourishment. Rushing from place to place, losing focus and connection, feeling overwhelmed, and eating on the run is no way to thrive. And striving to be super women leaves us with too much on our plate without the means to accomplish our goals.

One of the most healing things women can do is find ways to release stress, otherwise it bottles up inside and can negatively impact their mood, relationships, and choices. Once stress comes out to play, you won't feel so super, and feeling sexy, sensual, sensational, and savvy will likely be unattainable. Although we can't entirely avoid the daily stress in our lives, we can certainly take steps to relieve and release it and sometimes even cut it off at its source. If we don't, the stress will block our essential nourishment, causing us to relieve it in ways that don't serve us. This is why it's crucial to take on only what we can manage. Take it from me, this is a surefire way to offer stress an open invitation. Over time, the wiser me has learned to say no and be more mindful when saying yes.

My daughter and her college roommates coined an interesting term called FOMO (Fear of Missing Out). I have often felt this way, and, in recent years, have learned to listen to my inner self to squelch this tendency. It didn't happen until I was in my 40s. Thankfully, practicing yoga helped me gain the awareness I needed in order to say no. Like many things, this remains a work in progress.

Find Your Way Back

In times of stress, it is so easy to go off course. We must remember that now more than ever our warrior within thrives on flavorful foods that heal, calm, and nourish. Although sugar, alcohol, and caffeine may soothe, relax, or energize you in the short run, they won't serve you well. It's so much healthier to turn to yoga, meditation, journaling, or conversing with a good friend or partner.

Like many women who have reached their 50s, I know what it's like to lose yourself in grief and sadness. It permeates the present moment, is the thief of joy, compromises your health, and will impact your family. Even though you may have support of friends and family, it is vital that you find a lifeline. In my case, I am so grateful for the lifeline I found in yoga. The positive impact of this choice continues to this day because it helped me accept myself and discover the warrior in me.

"Yoga is not about self-improvement, it's about self-acceptance."

— Gurmukh Kaur Khalsa

Harness and Nourish Your Inner Guide

It's essential to remember to nourish your inner warrior when life is swirling around you like a kaleidoscope, and you feel like you've lost control. This is the time to harness your inner guidance and make the decision to show up as your best self. Nurture and nourish yourself. Taking one baby step to promote and preserve your well-being can lead you in the right direction. A gentle wave of inner calm will wash over you when you focus on what you can control. It's the simple things that reap the biggest benefits.

There are so many steps we can take each day to nourish our body, mind, heart, and soul. It can be as simple as:

- a glass of water or a nutritious meal
- a respite on a hammock or a good night's sleep
- a good book
- the touch of a loved one
- playing with your kids
- cooking, singing, dancing, painting, drawing, crafting
- a date night or a girl's night
- an energizing workout
- a barefoot walk on the grass or the beach

Always remember to be loving, kind, patient, and gentle with yourself.

Flourish Focus

"Food is a meditation, a sadhana, and a prayer. Good food is a virtue. Food can change your attitude, your behavior, your future, your present; it can change your health, wealth, happiness, everything."

— Yogi Bhajan

Self-Reflection:

What foods energize you and promote well-being?

_____

_____

_____

_____

_____

What activities make you smile and bring you joy, strength, and peace?

_____

_____

_____

_____

What warms your heart, speaks to your soul, and makes you feel alive?

_____

_____

_____

_____

Are your daily choices nourishing you?

_____

_____

_____

_____

What steps could you take to promote a healthier balance of real, life, and soul food?

_____

_____

_____

_____

> *"Stretching herself too thin,*
> *She breaks her connections.*
> *Staying too busy, she has no time.*
> *Doing for others, she neglects herself.*
> *Defining herself only through others,*
> *She loses her own definition.*
> *The wise woman waters her own garden first."*

— The Tao of Women'

Action Steps:

Real Food – Start your day with a healthy breakfast.

Life Food – Plan a time this week to engage in an activity that brings you joy and nourishment.

Soul Food – Make time every day to get quiet and still and listen to your inner voice.

Calm Heart Meditation *(courtesy of Laura Curran)*

1. Put your left hand on your heart and place your right hand up, palm facing forward, as if you were taking an oath.

2. Let the right elbow rest comfortably at your side.

3. On that right hand, gently connect the thumb tip to index-finger tip.

4. Close your eyes. Take a long, slow, deep breath in, and hold the breath in for as long as comfortable.

5. Slowly breathe out completely, and hold the breath out for as long as comfortable.

6. Keep taking those long, slow breaths, for 3–11 minutes.

Recipe: Power Up Chia Breakfast Pudding

Enjoy a nourishing start to your day.

Ingredients:

- 1 ½ cup coconut milk
- ⅓ cup raw cashews, soaked and rinsed
- 1 tsp pure vanilla extract
- 2 Tbsp organic maple syrup
- ⅓ cup whole chia seeds
- Berries and shredded coconut, for topping

Directions:

1. Blend coconut milk, cashews, vanilla, and maple syrup in a food processor or blender.
2. Pour into a glass jar.
3. Add chia seeds. Put lid on jar and shake.
4. Put in fridge. Shake again about an hour later.
5. Let chill and thicken overnight or at least three hours.
6. Take out and shake again. Add toppings and enjoy.

See more at https://nourishingsoulutions.com/power-up-chia-breakfast-pudding

Guiding Words from Flourish Contributor, Patsie Smith

Although I haven't met Patsie in person, I have had the pleasure of meeting her through the Soul Woman Sanctuary. She shares a deeply honest and inspiring story of survival in describing how she nourished herself back from darkness to a beautifully vibrant life.

—

As I reflect on the big 50 next year, I have absolutely no regrets because however imperfect my experiences have been, they were stepping-stones toward the complete and whole person I am today. My life journey was challenging. Due to a dysfunctional childhood, I entered adolescent and teenage years confused, struggling, and very lost. My inability to navigate through life was like an internal tumor in my psyche that grew until it exploded in my face at 21. Weary and having lost all will to continue, I overdosed on pharmaceutical tablets and tried to end the torture. I was exhausted from battling life as a victim.

Amazingly, I survived, and it was the turning point of my life. I explored forms of natural healing and spiritual wisdom and experienced the ups and downs of self-discovery. I also depended on alcohol to help numb the emotions that were too intense for me to confront. Dredging up my old hurts, pains, and fears was tumultuous because it meant confronting all my demons. It took every ounce of my courage and hard work to reprogram my brain, release my pent-up emotions, heal my weary body, and to reveal my true essence.

Following my self-healing and transformation, I ended my abusive relationship with alcohol and focused on replen-

ishing my liver and body with natural foods and herbs. Meditations and spiritual wisdom connected me to my true essence and anchored me in peace. Through that anchor, nature activities, yoga, dancing, and drumming slowly helped me to heal and restructure my reality. The more I healed, the more my wholeness was restored.

Nature is life essence itself. Being with and submerging in nature always replenished me with a silent strength. Yoga was a dynamic meditation, for it took me fully into the present moment while releasing blockages in my physical body through postures and breathwork.

Today I look back at my journey with gratitude and wisdom. Out of my healings, and blossoming from a caterpillar into a butterfly, I now thrive in this amazing life with joy and passion. Every day is special because I guide others on their healing journeys. The ancient Eastern wisdom of being accepting, flexible, adaptable, and open resonates with me. I naturally look forward to the coming years with an adventurous, open spirit. I embrace every dream, vision, and possibility. Life isn't just about a beginning or an end and the changes in between. It's about being fully in the present moment with peace and acceptance, which leads us into ageless vibrancy and joy.

CHAPTER 5

Celebrating You

You may or may not know that there are perks that accompany each coming year. One of the biggest ones is a sense of self-worth. As a young girl, I was afraid to raise my hand to answer a question or even to get ice cream. It was challenging to express myself in a serious matter without breaking into tears. Thankfully, with each passing year my confidence grew. My Mom really helped draw me out through conversation, humor, understanding, and a love of children's literature. She was a gifted teacher with an uncanny ability to bring forth the best in children.

I remember an adorable book titled, *"I can't said the ant."* This whimsical rhyming story describes a sweet little powerless ant who doesn't know how to help the teapot after she has an accident, but with the encouragement of the kitchen residents, she emerges as the teapot's hero. So, whenever I said, "I can't," my Mom's reply was, "You must, said the crust, I can't bear it, said the carrot," and other phrases from the story. This helped me to laugh at myself and instilled a sense of confidence in me. *Amelia Bedelia* was another character that my Mom used to relieve my fear of mistakes since this confused maid mixed up everything from dusting the furniture to dressing the chicken. She took everything literally, but no matter what the antics, *Amelia Bedelia* was fine in the end.

The Role of a Lifetime

After giving birth to my babies, my confidence took a big leap forward. Perhaps this was because I always yearned to be a mom, and I felt so content in this role. Having the opportunity to focus on my babies instead of myself empowered me to advocate for myself and voice my opinion. I know some women struggle with the transition to motherhood, but for me it felt like the role of a lifetime, what I was meant for, and this was the first time in my life that I felt really good at something right down to my core. I discovered the intuition I didn't know I had, learned to trust and follow my instincts, and truly relaxed into being a mom. While other women worried if their babies were getting enough milk, I just knew that my breasts were fully nourishing them. When they woke at night, I didn't worry, and typically they just went back to sleep.

> *"Birth is not only about making babies. Birth is about making mothers - strong, competent, capable mothers who trust themselves and know their inner strength."*

— Barbara Katz Rothman

Experience Offers a Stronger Sense of Self

Our experiences impact our choices, change the course of our lives, and hopefully make us more resilient. I found this to be true as I recovered from the tragic death of my brother where I really felt like I lost a part of me to grief. One of the hardest things about losing special people is that we have one less person to share our triumphs, joy, and sorrows with in life. It was difficult to reconcile life without him, but I had to make the choice to journey back. When I found a healthier me, I discovered a deeper connection to my soul. I grew more decisive and gained clarity and awareness, which helped me to address my needs and to discern what and who served my best interests.

Be Grateful

Experiencing loss is inevitable as we grow older, but I can say that losing Joey, my best friend, Sue, and many other special people along the way has fueled my zest for life and makes me appreciate each and every day. As a Health Coach, this motivates me to guide women on a nourishing path to embrace vibrant living.

Although we all have different experiences that change us, with each passing decade we grow into our true essence. We learn what our gifts really are, and sometimes they surprise us since they may have been the very things we tried to hide as younger women.

Connecting to Ourselves

The glory of stepping into the next season is that we find our way back to ourselves and learn that we are enough. We come to believe in ourselves at a much deeper level, so we no longer need to pretend or hide what we once deemed flaws since we can accept our whole package. At this age, we recognize that no one is perfect, that we all have challenges that shape the way we look and feel, and that we all have gifts to share. Even though my confidence blossomed a little more with each decade, there are still moments where I yearn for it. This awareness helps us advocate for our own well-being and celebrate who we really are... and that's priceless.

So go ahead and "friend" yourself. Have a love affair with you and cherish all that you are. The most important relationship you can have is with yourself, so if you haven't spent much time focusing on you, it's time because all relationships are born out of this one.

Sometimes younger women try to be everything to everyone, and over time, this really does exact a toll. That was my experience since I was a bit of a people pleaser and wanted to like everyone and have them like me. My decisions were often based on what others wanted. I was comfortable with serving the needs of others while often ignoring my own.

> *"When a woman becomes her own best friend,*
> *life is easier."*

— Diane Von Furstenberg

Treat Yourself Better

As women, we are often are too hard on ourselves. If you haven't already evolved beyond this behavior, now is the time to start treating yourself like your own best friend. Obviously, this is still a work in progress for me and may be for you as well. When you find yourself engaging in self-sabotage, remember to shower yourself with love and kindness just like you would someone special because that's what you are. It's paramount to make choices that honor yourself and focus on friends, family, and lovers who honor and celebrate you, too.

As women, we must learn to celebrate ourselves. When we do this, it resonates with friends, lovers, and family— who then champion us as well. Having special people to share your bliss, celebrate your success, and support you in times of need is so important. You'll notice who your real friends are in times of sadness or turmoil because they stick around. These are the people who really matter. Likewise, it's essential to give as much as you get.

You Get What You Give

At different points in our lives, we may yearn for people to celebrate our strides and share in our life. Don't be dissuaded if they don't do it right away— just think of this as a reshuffle and start showing up in other people's lives to celebrate them. Soon, special people will appear to share in your life. Celebration is a two way street, so don't be afraid to invite people in.

Instead of focusing on what you deem to be failures, focus on the strides you are achieving in life. These are the building blocks for success. No need to get hung up on failures since this just stresses us, diminishes our self worth, and interferes with enjoying the present moment.

Take Time to Reconnect

Do you ever wonder why you maintain friendships with some people while losing touch with very special friends? Sometimes, it's circumstantial, but often it's because you really didn't know yourself so well, weren't aware of your needs, and weren't able to discern who really mattered. It's never too late to reach out to someone special in your life. One thing I love about social media is that it offers the opportunity to reunite with special friends or relatives. I am so grateful for the reconnected friendships that have blossomed in this way.

Dump the Drama

Life experience affords us the opportunity to move away from or resolve unhealthy relationships while shining a beautiful light on ourselves, our needs, and the people we want to dance with through life. With our well-earned wisdom, we can do it so much better the second time around. Although we can't relive our past, we can focus on gathering with those who make our heart and soul smile.

"You can't start the next chapter of your life if you keep re-reading or trying to re-write the last one."

— Author Unknown

As you evolve through life, you'll notice that you aren't afraid to show who you are. You don't waste time trying to conform or fit in like younger women sometimes do.

You understand your needs, can be of support to your friends, and are more apt to value and cultivate healthy relationships. It takes courage to be who you really are and to voice what you value. When you stand up and show up, you'll attract more meaningful relationships because this deepens your connection to authentic souls.

Bring Your Relationships Into Focus

It's uplifting to be surrounded by people who you really care about since spending time with superficial friends can stir up loneliness. This goes for family members, too. Even when a relationship is lacking substance, look for a way to carve out a more mean-ingful one. Little reminders or prompts can go a long way with your immediate family. There are also times when intimacy may be reduced to a minimum or might be missing altogether, but as a confident woman, you have the option to nurture and create more intimacy with your lover.

Likewise, we occasionally need to reassess our friend-ships, so we can carve out new ones, while letting go of those that no longer serve us. Just like cleansing our bodies from toxins, cleaning our homes, and servicing our cars, sometimes our relationships need to be purged to make room for the relationships that truly nourish us.

Surround yourself with people who love, support, encourage, inspire, and celebrate you as well as those who make you feel happy, desired, and welcome.

Flourish Focus

"The older I get ... the more comfortable I am in my own beautiful skin. What I once thought were flaws ... are now what I choose to celebrate."

— Author Unknown

Self-Reflection:

Jot down at least three things that you celebrate about yourself.

_____

_____

_____

_____

Who celebrates you and makes you feel happy?

_____

_____

_____

_____

Action Step: Do something special to celebrate yourself, like buying a beautiful floral bouquet.

List some ideas here:

_____

_____

_____

Recipe: Ravishing Raw Cashew Cheese Cupcakes

Nothing says celebrate better than a delicious cupcake or a glass of Champagne.

Quantity varies depending on size of cupcake pan.

Makes 30 mini cupcakes using a silicone cupcake container. You can also use small freezable glass bowls. Do not use an aluminum or metal pan.

If you have extra, you can use it as a yummy cashew coconut cream dipping sauce for fruit.

Ingredients:

- 1 cup macadamia nuts
- 1½ cups cashews
- ¼ cup pitted Medjool dates
- ¼ cup dried coconut flakes
- ⅓ cup coconut oil, melted (*when the oil is gently warmed it turns to liquid*)
- ¼ cup lime juice or juice of 1 freshly squeezed lime
- ¼ cup raw honey
- 1 tsp pure vanilla extract
- ⅓ cup water
- 1 cup mixed berries (*blueberries, strawberries, blackberries, and raspberries*)

Directions:

1. Place macadamia nuts in large bowl and cover with cold water. Place cashews in separate bowl and cover with cold water. Soak nuts for four hours, then rinse, drain, and set aside.
2. Pulse macadamia nuts and dates in food processor to a sticky crumb-like consistency.
3. Press macadamia nut mixture into silicone mini cupcake pan, about 1 tsp per mini cup. You can also add some coconut flakes here. This makes up your crust.
4. Place cashews, coconut oil, lime juice, and raw honey in the bowl of a food processor. Add in pure vanilla extract, gradually add in water, and purée until smooth.
5. Pour mixture onto crust in cupcake pan, sprinkle with dried coconut flakes and freeze 1–2 hours, or until firm.
6. Remove from freezer, scoop out onto a plate, top with berries, and serve.

See more at https://www.nourishingsoulutions.com/ravishing-raw-cashew-cheese-cupcakes/

Guiding Words from Flourish Contributor, Liz Murray

I had the pleasure of meeting Liz via a virtual program. As a holistic health coach, Liz has a beautiful way of celebrating herself, living vibrantly, and empowering other women to flourish.

—

Each decade has a theme and a life skill to learn. My 20s were about becoming an adult woman, navigating the corporate world (ugh!), and learning how to be in relationships with others. My 30s were about marriage, understanding my core essence, and building a life with my husband. My 40s were about motherhood and learning to forgive. And now, I am in my 50s in the midst of learning and experiencing this decade, and I see some themes emerging...

Body: I spent most of my life hating my body, trying to diet, exercise, and starve myself into a physical version of me that would somehow be acceptable, but I couldn't handle it for long and would binge, sometimes for days. I was at war with this one precious body. In my 50s, I now know that I will never diet again. It doesn't serve me. I have made peace with my imperfections. My belly is soft; it grew a baby and is the seat of my intuition. I now focus on nourishing myself accordingly. Eating delicious, healthy food, moving my body in pleasurable ways, and dressing myself so I feel beautiful are my guiding forces. Leafy greens, walks in the woods, and yoga have replaced the frozen "diet" food and boot-camp exercise classes.

Career: I spent years trying to fit into someone else's mold. I wore suits and pantyhose and carried a briefcase, as if playing a role in a soul-sucking job I was ill-suited for. Most people who meet me now can't believe I lived this way for ten years. What freedom I have now! I get to help amazing women transform their lives! My work life and "real" life are gorgeously intertwined. When my clients put their trust in me by investing in themselves, it is so humbling, and I feel immense gratitude— a much different experience from simply getting a paycheck.

Relationships: I was so caught up in the game of "you make me feel" ... and I see now that relationships exist to teach me about myself. They are a mirror. If I am experiencing a strong negative reaction toward someone else, it is time to shine the light inward, as these are really unacceptable feelings toward myself.

My 50s have been about self-love and self-acceptance. The essence of a life well-lived is love. Love of self, love of others, our families and dear friends, and the animals that depend on us and our beautiful planet. In closing, here is a quote by my favorite author, Mary Oliver...

"You do not have to be good.
You do not have to walk on your knees for a hundred miles through the desert, repenting.
You only have to let the soft animal of your body love what it loves."

CHAPTER 6

Finding and Filling Your Fountain of Youth

Who doesn't want to find a fountain of youth? There are lots of commercials, magazine ads, and infomercials selling us this magical destination in the form of miracle potions and creams. Although I enjoy select skin care products, supplements, super foods, healing foods, and essential oils that promote vitality, you just can't beat the benefits of play, pleasure, laughter, and love. The truth is simple: your fountain of youth is right inside you. It's in your dreams, your mindset, your attitudes, and your desires. You just need to feed it. Once you rediscover these youthful benefits, you'll be ready to embrace them every day.

"Taking joy in living is a woman's best cosmetic."

— Rosalind Russell

The Power of Play

We can easily forget just how fun it is to play and all too often believe we grow out of this basic need. Here's a little secret– playing isn't just for kids, especially if you are a women seeking ageless vibrancy.

Remember not wanting the day to end when you were called home for dinner? I still feel like that! When I was little, play dates were nonexistent. We just went out, called our friends, and played. I have fond memories of digging in my yard, making forts in the woods, riding waves, collecting seashells and building sand castles, playing roller derby, pool, board games, Red Light Green Light, and hide and go seek. I'm sure you can add to this list.

When we look back, the things we were drawn to as children are the very things that truly nourish us today. When we rediscover these favorite pastimes, they are often the gifts we share with others or the things that soothe our soul. For example, although I no longer play with dolls, I loved playing with my babies, and instead of teaching dolls, I teach women to nourish their way to a vibrant life. An evening or day at the beach, bike riding, and swimming still bring me joy. I used to write stories, and I now love writing my nourishing news and was inspired to write this book. I fell in love with my Betty Crocker oven and now love cooking up nourishing and scrumptious recipes, and I enjoy teaching women to do the same. When we revisit what we enjoyed in our past, we unleash our creativity and maximize our joy.

Fitness Should Feel Good

Think about how relaxed your body feels after some serious play time. All that running, jumping, throwing, and laughing keeps your body flowing and fills your fountain. It nourishes your body, offers a vacation for your mind, and can melt your stress away. The more we enjoy ourselves, the more youthful we feel. So invite that little girl inside you out to play!

Women often put fitness on the bottom of their list because they don't engage in it enough to experience the benefits . Sometimes you find blessings as a result of an injury. This was the case for me when I broke my knee in my 20s and was disabled for six months. I never took my body for granted again, and my determination to restore my knee offered me a life-long appreciation for consistent exercise. It's essential to embrace and engage in activities that bring you joy, otherwise it just feels like another chore. Fitness needs to be fun.

A playful mindset can transform your life. Maybe exercise feels like a chore to you. Perhaps a gym membership won't work for you, but if you get reacquainted with the action packed activities of your youth, you will find a playful outlet for fitness and fun that ignites you. Likewise, if you have an adventurous spirit, set your sights on activities that inspire you. One of my new favorites is Stand-up Paddle Boarding. I'm not much of a gym rat, but I love yoga, swimming and running on the beach. Yoga offers the perfect balance of stillness and movement that my body craves. It truly nourishes my body, mind, and soul.

"Exercise should be about rewarding your body with strength, movement, and the feel good release of endorphins, not punishing your body for food that you have eaten or weight that you haven't been able to release."

— Marc David

Play's Best Friend – Pleasure

Pleasure is closely related to play but is perhaps a bit more alluring. Pleasure puts a smile on your face, a warm feeling in your heart, and makes you feel good. If you invite her, she'll join you. She's never met guilt since pleasure doesn't have regrets. She lives in the present moment intent on experiencing life's indulgences. We can reach out for pleasure every day. It all depends on how you define it. You'll find it in a good morning kiss or a delicious treat, by cuddling with a sweet baby or lover, taking a walk on the beach, enjoying a deep massage or a scrumptious meal, diving into a wave, spending a night out with friends and dancing to your favorite tunes, wearing your favorite dress, sitting on top of a mountain, sleeping peacefully, or relaxing on a hammock. The possibilities are endless.

Pleasure doesn't need permission or an appointment, but if she's been scarce be sure to invite her to fill your fountain. Pleasure doesn't recognize age, rules, or limits. That's why it is an essential ingredient of vibrant living.

Keep Filling Your Fountain

You will thrive with a pleasure filled lifestyle and stagnate with one based on deprivation. Many women have the misguided belief that adhering to a strict diet and exercise regimen will fuel their fountain of youth. They are comfortable with restriction and don't make room for pleasure. This joyless path may keep them thin and fit but at what cost? This mindset won't fill their fountain of youth and could actually cause it to dry up.

The Beauty of Laughter

Laughter and love are best friends with pleasure and play, and they all feed your fountain of youth and help you flourish. Just think about how young you feel after a fun night of laughs. Whenever I call my mom and step dad, all I hear is laughter. That really keeps them young at heart. And when I participated and presented at a Flourish Fest in Ireland last year, I loved how they described a fun night, "We had such good craic."

Try your best to find something to laugh about every day. It is soothing to the soul, nourishing to the heart, and does wonders for a woman's youthful vitality. It also relieves stress, one of the #1 hindrances to vibrancy. And when you glance in a mirror, you may even see a younger you since laughing offers quite a beauty boost. You would be surprised how much a lack of laughter and joy ages us. When I view photos of myself during the period when I was grieving my brother's loss, I look 10 years older.

Laughter promotes vitality in numerous ways:
(visit https://www.laughteryoga.org/english/home)

- Boosts libido
- Calms, relaxes, and relieves the symptoms of stress
- Lowers cortisol levels
- Promotes a younger look
- Revs up your metabolism
- Boosts serotonin – the feel good hormone
- Increases endorphins
- Promotes a healthy heart and immune system

"All You Need Is Love"

Love is an essential ingredient for flourishing women. Vitamin L nourishes us deeply. It comes in many forms, so everyone can find it in their lives whether it's self-love, spousal love, intimate love, Momma love, love of children, love for a pet, love of family, girl friend love, or brotherly love. And guess who you have to love first? You – of course. If you don't love yourself up, you won't be able to nurture anyone else. So start by loving and accepting yourself.

Of course, a gratifying love life is something to strive for, but we need all types of love to flourish. We are beings that need to give, feel, and share. The more ways you can find to engage in loving activities the better. Whether it's caring for others, gathering with friends, intimate moments, writing love letters, holding hands, looking in your lover's eyes, celebrating with family, helping friends and family, supporting someone in need, caring for animals, or volunteering your services, make sure that love fills your heart because your fountain of youth is thirsty.

"Inside every child is an 'emotional tank' waiting to be filled with love."

— Gary Chapman, The Five Love Languages

It's Important to Say It

We can easily overlook how important it is to say and hear these three little words, "I love you." They feel good to say and hear, and the more you do it the happier the people around you will be. Without it, we really are just empty vessels. Even in loving relationships, we can easily get disconnected. Anyone who has been married for a long time knows that while embracing the peaks you also have to love your way out of the valleys. It is ever so important to tell our lovers how much they mean to us as well as anyone else we care about.

Love is expressed in a variety of ways, and we each have a way that feels most comfortable. Check out The Five Languages of Love to gain a greater understanding of how people show and receive love.

"Let us be grateful to people who make us happy, they are the charming gardeners who make our souls blossom."

— Marcel Proust

Replenish Your Fountain

Your lifestyle directly impacts your fountain. Your level of fitness, hours of sleep, the food and beverages you consume, and your ability to relieve stress all play a key role. In fact, Dr. Mark Hyman says sugar affects your fountain,

"[It] reduces your growth hormone (GH) production. *(GH) is your "fountain of youth" hormone that you mostly produce during deep sleep. Secreted by the pituitary gland, GH improves muscle mass, helps your body utilize fat, and helps maintain optimal libido. Reduced muscle mass, increased abdominal obesity and risk for Type 2 diabetes, and lower libido are hallmark symptoms of GH deficiencies. Researchers find a direct link between GH, insulin levels, and sexual function. Studies show insulin reduces your body's ability to make (GH), altering testosterone levels and reducing libido."*

Your fountain of youth also refills or depletes based on how your activities, food, choices, interactions, and responsibilities make you feel. Success, achievement, happiness, pleasure, praise, joy, gratitude, intimacy, contentment, peace, connection, and service fill your fountain, whereas difficult relationships and circumstances, stress, conflict, grief, illness, and sadness deplete your fountain.

"Your body naturally makes less GH as you age. No debate. At the same time, let's stop blaming everything on age: when GH decreases, you grow older. That puts you in the driver's seat: you have a sacred opportunity to turn your sinking vessel around and keep GH in the happy zone."

— Dr. Sara Gottfried

A Mantra to Self-Assess

My kids often mimic me by saying, "How does that make you feel?" No matter what happens, good or bad, I always ask this question — so much so that they often beat me to the punch. The funny thing is that I thought this question was my own because assessing and sharing our feelings can be so healing. Then one day I shared some exciting news with my Mom, and her reply was, "That must have made you feel good." I burst into laughter because now I knew just where that mantra came from, and I won't be surprised if my children continue it.

Take notice when you are feeling happy, energized, and youthful. Likewise, consider how old you feel when your energy is depleted. Last year, my husband took me to Bermuda to ring in my 50th, and we felt so revitalized from enjoying ourselves and each other. This fabulous celebration made us both feel like we were 20 again. We even look younger in our trip photos! It's amazing how relaxation, intimacy, pleasure, and joy can truly replenish your fountain. So go out and enjoy yourself, eat healthy and delicious food, get a good night's sleep, and feel your fountain fill up.

Flourish Focus

Self-Reflection:

> "We are all little girls in aging bodies. No matter how old we are, we are still that little girl that skipped rope, roller skated on the sidewalk, skinned knees, wore braids with barrettes or ribbons, and ate ice cream bars from the ice cream man…"

> — Jo Schlehofer

Write down 3–5 activities you enjoyed as a young girl. Do you enjoy these now in some way? How does it feel when you engage in these activities? If you enjoy new activities, what are they? How do they make you feel?

_____

_____

_____

_____

_____

_____

_____

_____

_____

_____

_____

_____

_____

Action Steps:

1. Get in touch with the playful child inside and participate in activities that are fun, feel good, and make you laugh.

   _____

   _____

   _____

2. If your fitness regimen feels like a chore, stop immediately and find a nourishing activity that you enjoy which makes you feel good and offers you some pleasure.

   _____

   _____

   _____

Recipe: Satiating Super Food Chocolate Berry Sorbet

What's more pleasure-filled than a dose of luscious dark chocolate ice cream, or, in this case, a satiating chocolate sorbet?

Ingredients:

- ½ cup pure water
- 2 Tbsp maca
- ½ cup raw honey
- 1 tsp vanilla
- ½ cup raw cacao powder
- 1 cup frozen raspberries
- 1 cup goji berries

Directions:

1. If you don't have a Vitamix, thaw the fruit for several minutes to
   make it easier to blend.
2. Add all ingredients to blender and blend until smooth.
3. Enjoy this scrumptious and indulgent treat immediately
   or freeze in ice cube trays for a frozen dessert.
4. Decorate with flaked coconut.

See more at https://www.nourishingsoulutions.com/satiating-super-food-chocolate-berry-sorbet/

Guiding Words from Flourish Contributor, Jayne Justice

Although Jayne and I studied together at the Institute for Integrative Nutrition, we didn't meet until a mutual friend set us up to be roommates for a nutrition conference. We became fast friends and enjoyed each other's zest for life. Jayne is well suited for health coaching and is a beautiful example of a woman who has discovered her fountain of youth.

—

I am a woman of strong character, hard work, grace, success, and beauty with a bit of stubbornness thrown in. As each birthday rolls around, my goal has always been to maintain or surpass my level of health and fitness. As I approach 58, I reflect on where I am, where I am going, how I feel, and how I look! After all, we are women and looking good is important, but how I FEEL is more important. Reflecting on years past, I humbly acknowledge my accomplishments and mistakes and realize I have more life to live.

Living a vibrant, joyous life is my gift to myself. I deserve it. I want to wake up every day feeling good, both physically and mentally. Life has become more and more about BEING not DOING. Being my authentic self, living my truth, enjoying each day, and realizing this is ENOUGH.

As a young teenager, I loved playing baseball with my brothers, jumping into the creek from a rope, as well as being a girly girl. My mother had a huge influence on me. As we watched the Miss America pageant every year, she would say, "You can do that. You will be Miss America some day." And I never doubted her, so when I was crowned Miss Missouri 1977, it was the most exciting point in my life. Having achieved that dream and going on to the Miss America pageant was thrilling. Winning the swimsuit competition was a testament to my focus on fitness, so much so that I went on to study nutrition and major in dietetics in college.

But working as a Dietician in a hospital was not my passion; motivating, teaching, and coaching others to BE healthy NOW was. When I eventually settled in California, I found my nirvana, met my husband, and gave birth to a beautiful baby girl in my 40s. The challenges of infertility and pregnancy changed my perspective on health and life, and I was drawn toward a new career as a holistic health coach.

Today, I enjoy Bikram yoga, Pilates, 5 Rhythms dance, walking on the beach, ocean swims, and kickboxing. Meditation, quiet times, listening to music, and playing the piano also fuel my soul. My favorite affirmation is 'I am good enough.'

I would tell my younger self to let go of fear, to live in the moment, to play more and think less, and to laugh more and harder. Life is truly a journey. I am grateful for this path and this wisdom. I am a bit more patient, know myself better, and am calmer and happier.

Today is the gift. Wrap it in as pretty a package as you can.

CHAPTER 7

Discovering the Sweetness in Life

How often do you stop to think about how sweet
life really is? No matter what is going on in your life,
you can always find some sweetness. Now mind you,
I don't mean sweet foods like candy and cookies. I
am talking about sweet moments like taking in a
gorgeous sunset with your lover, watching your son
surf or a toddler play, diving into a wave or enjoying
a scenic bike ride, laughing with a group of special
friends and making someone smile, cuddling up in
bed with your husband and kids, enjoying a delicious
meal with your family, nursing your baby, planting
flowers, playing music, singing, and the list goes on.

Over time, our life experiences can make us feel bitter
if we let them and no amount of sugar will satisfy
the hunger of a bitter heart. It's not always easy, but
by releasing these feelings you will also let go of the

need to feed them with sugar. When you find yourself ruminating, observe any thoughts of bitterness and dissuade them with sweet memories and thoughts.

"The purpose of life, after all, is to live it, to taste experience to the utmost, to reach out eagerly and without fear for newer and richer experience."

— Eleanor Roosevelt

Don't be Seduced by Sugar

Sweet cravings can occur when you are thirsty, tired, hungry, upset, sad, frustrated, nervous, stressed, angry, or not consuming enough protein, fats, or essential nutrients. There's no denying that a sugar fix makes us feel good in the moment, and there is nothing wrong with enjoying treats on occasion, as long as you choose mindfully and enjoy them. I don't eat a lot of cake, but for my birthday, I so enjoy a scrumptious piece of German chocolate cake with whipped cream frosting. I am worthy of this delight and don't beat myself up for what others may deem an undeserving indulgence. Have you ever chosen the salad when you really wanted a tastier meal? I just encouraged a client to mindfully enjoy her celebratory anniversary dinner rather than depriving herself to compensate for a recent indulgence. That is no way to treat yourself and will result in bitterness and increased cravings for sugar.

Just like a sweet talking guy, sugar knows how to seduce you. But after that fix is over and your energy levels plummet, you'll be seeking another fix to sustain you. Make no mistake – sugar is addictive, and its impact worsens over time, so reign in the sugar and replace it with nourishing things that really serve you. It really is essential to consistently get a good night's rest, nourish yourself with nutritious foods, keep yourself hydrated, and engage in activities that relieve stress and enhance your mood if you want to steer clear of sugar. And when you get off the sugar roller coaster, you'll avoid the problematic mood swings and fuel yourself with the sweetness that surrounds you.

And as we mature, we can easily succumb to the desire for sweets, sometimes indulging to fill a void, such as boredom or loneliness; however, refined sugar can easily reek havoc on our immune system, hormones, monthly cycle, weight, energy levels, skin, blood sugar, and ability to sleep, and can also increase the risk of cancer, diabetes, and heart disease. Did you know that processed sugar can even increase hot flashes?

In your search for a sweet life you may be looking in all the wrong places:

- Finding comfort in sugary, fatty, and salty snacks.
- Fueling your body with caffeine to make it through each day.
- Relying on alcohol to relax you.

Discovering Your Own Sweet Spot

If you have an insatiable desire for sweets, then it's time to sweeten up your life with sensational activities and people. You'll discover how much better you'll feel when you trade the sugary treats for a sweet life. If you are ready to reclaim your zest for life, then it's time to discover your sweet spot. This is a personal place filled with exuberance, joy, and connection. It's your happy place where you feel at ease and in sync. Let your unique interests guide you toward the sweetness that makes your heart smile.

"I still find each day too short for all the thoughts I want to think, all the walks I want to take, all the food I want to eat, all the books I want to read, and all the friends I want to see."

— John Burroughs

When your life is feeling bland, it's time to seek out adventure and embrace activities that excite and fulfill you. Last year, I discovered an enticing Flourish Fest Retreat in Ireland and felt called to attend and even wound up being a retreat presenter as well as a participant. My sister joined me, and we fully embraced our Irish adventure.

But an adventure doesn't necessarily require a lot of thought, maps, and travel plans. It can be as simple as taking a walk somewhere you haven't been before. I love finding little hideaways in my neighborhood. Asking a new friend to join you can make it even more of an adventure. I've been riding my bike, jogging, and cross-country skiing in a park near me for years, then one beautiful spring day I asked a new friend to join me for a walk. We went off the path and found a beautiful little beach on a lake that I hadn't even realized was there. Now this was a sweet moment that we both enjoyed! It was certainly much tastier than a few cookies.

"A wise friend told me that your fifties can be the time you discover what freedom means for you. And she was right."

— Amy Hempel

Life is made up of delicious moments. It's up to us to discover them since finding the sweet spot in everyday life is a beautiful way to cultivate with a taste for vibrant living.

Flourish Focus

"What grace to be alive and know the day in all its sweetness."

— Ram Dass

Self-Reflection:

How can you make each day of your life sweeter?

_____

_____

_____

_____

Describe where you were and how you felt when you were recently in touch with your sweet spot.

_____

_____

_____

_____

Where do you feel most alive, free, and in sync?

_____

_____

_____

_____

Action Steps:

1. Plan a simple adventure for yourself.
   List some ideas:

   _____

   _____

   _____

   _____

   _____

2. Satisfy your sugar cravings with seasonal
   sweet fruits and vegetables.

   - Berries
   - Bananas
   - Watermelon
   - Cantaloupe
   - Carrots
   - Sweet potatoes
   - Beets

Recipe: Nutty Banana Delight

Sometimes we just need a sweet treat.

Ingredients:

- 4 bananas
- ½ cup almonds, crushed or ground*
- ½ cup walnuts, crushed or ground*
- ½ cup coconut flakes
- ½ cup raw cacao

you can use any nuts—cashews and pistachios, for example

Directions:

1. Mix almonds, walnuts, coconut flakes, and raw cacao together in a bowl.
2. Slice each banana into thin slices and dip in mixture.
3. Place in a flat container and freeze.

See more at https://www.nourishingsoulutions.com/nutty-banana-delights/

Guiding Words from Flourish Contributor, Samyak Yamauchi

I had the good fortune of meeting Samyak via the virtual world. As a retired teacher of 30 years and presently an artist/soul-work facilitator, Samyak has an interesting and inspiring message about discovering her sweet spot in life.

—

I'm very fortunate. I'm coming to the end of my third year of retirement and am in good health in a good relationship. I don't have to go anywhere. I don't have to do anything. I get to paint every day. It's like being on a permanent vacation.

Right after I retired, my husband and I took a seven-week road trip. We saw beautiful land, spent time with good people, and it was fun and exciting. When I returned, a friend asked me, "What did you learn?" No one had ever asked me that before. My answer was, "I learned how noisy the world is and how hard it is to find silence."

I found it in the cliffs and canyons in Utah and on the mesa tops in New Mexico, but once home I couldn't find it. My life was noisy. More importantly, I couldn't find silence in myself. My mind was constantly full of too many words and ideas. But a couple years later, I slipped into the silence.
I let LOVE into my heart one night. Just like that – I just let it in. There, I found the sweet spot where silence surrounds with calm understanding and acceptance of what IS.

The events that happen in my life are noisy distractions that manifest themselves in order to remind me to stay

*in the space of silence and peace. These events rise up ...
I meet them, breathe them, let them go, and return to
my center.*

*Recently, important things, big things shook me up and
out of the silence. My sister died an unexpected and
difficult death. I was shocked and so saddened. She
died just days after I found out how very sick she was.
I've watched four members of my immediate family
die. I've listened to each of them take their final breath
in and release it out. I've felt the silence that follows as
the spirit leaves the body. It's a stillness that makes me
aware of the silence that exists in me.*

*Next, I closed the book on a friendship that was going
nowhere. I had held onto that friendship even though
it didn't feed my soul until, while painting, I saw the
truth. I found silence in letting go. And in the most
destructive noise of all, knowing of a friend's drug
addiction and being unable to do anything about it, I
have found silence in accepting that I don't know what
will happen next.*

*As the shock, sadness, and grief of these events is dissi-
pating, my husband and I went to the beach to accompany our granddaughter's first grade class on a field
trip. The weather was good. It was fun to see all the
little kids having fun. It was fun to walk on the beach,
sleep in a motel, go out to eat, and spend time with our
family.*

*What did I learn? I learned that life is really noisy,
and it's hard to find silence — but you can. It's just
that it might be found in places you wouldn't think to
look. As I emerged from these challenging awakening
experiences, I slipped into what I had been looking for
my whole life — the spiritual sweet spot of knowing who
I truly am.*

CHAPTER 8

Weaving in Harmony

Harmony is a key ingredient in a flourishing life, and even though it doesn't mean that your life is without challenges and in perfect balance, it means that life is flowing in the right direction, and that your goals, daily tasks, and activities are in alignment.

> *"Be like a flower, beautiful in essence,*
> *rooted in being!"*

— Mary Byrne, Garden of Pensiveness

It's vital to strive for harmony in all aspects of your life because your stress level, career, finances, relationship, and spiritual connection all play an essential role. When we feel stressed or off kilter, it's often because something in our life needs attention.

Stress can easily set off a chain reaction disrupting our sense of harmony. At Integrative Nutrition, Joshua Rosenthal introduced the Circle of Life exercise as a way to achieve balance and well-being.

Seven Key Areas

- Family
- Friendship
- Wellness: health, nutrition, fitness, stress, and sleep
- Intimacy
- Spirituality/Faith/Connection
- Purpose: career, hobbies, volunteer activities
- Finances

When one of these seven areas is undernourished, there's a tendency to fill a void by overcompensating in another area. Here are some common scenarios:

- Ongoing and unresolved stress within the family or in the workplace compromises your health and causes you to overcompensate in other areas and turn to unhealthy habits to soothe these feelings (i.e. problems at home may cause you to spend more time at work as a way to avoid the situation).

- A tragic loss or life-altering injury or disease can easily turn your life upside down.

- Women may focus too critically on their jobs, children, friends, or turn to food, excessive spending, and self-medicating with drugs or alcohol when intimacy is lacking.

- When women lack a sense of purpose, they may also turn to food or alcohol and focus excessively on their family or on trivial matters.

Identify Imbalances

It's important to check in with yourself to see where you can infuse some energy and focus on releasing the blockages you are feeling. When you discover discord, it's time to address the gaps and guide yourself back to center. I have found that practicing yoga regularly is like a GPS for the soul, offering a greater ability to identify and resolve misalignment. It truly helps me gain awareness, get to the heart of the matter, and feel more aligned.

Slow Down and Nourish Yourself

You may have learned by now that one of the best ways to promote hormone harmony and well-being is by slowing your pace and scheduling some down time. You don't always realize it, but when you run on empty you starve your body of nourishment in so many ways. I have had to teach myself to be mindful of this because I often find myself with an overflowing plate of obligations, responsibilities, and activities. I have seen how this compromises my immune system, lowers my libido, and frazzles me. A clear schedule, enjoying some R & R, embracing family and friends, beach walks, ocean swims, yoga, and beautiful bike rides relax me and offer a refreshing libido boost.

"The psyches and souls of women also have their own cycles and seasons of doing and solitude, running and staying, being involved and being removed, questing and resting, creating and incubating, being of the world and returning to the soul-place."

— Clarissa Pinkola Estés

Since I am always searching for effective wellness resources and tools, I found Young Living Essential Oils to be an outstanding complement to a healthy lifestyle. They promote everyday wellness in numerous ways, and specific oils can restore energy and help balance your hormones. Learn more at http://judygriffin.marketingscents.com/goland13

Although harmony is a work in progress, when we weave it in one layer at a time we feel calmer, content, and connected to our essence. This plays a major role in our well-being as it promotes hormone balance, makes us less susceptible to illness, nourishes us at a deep level, and helps our body work for us. Everyone needs to engage in respites that restore, replenish, and revitalize. Find pleasure in the paradise you create. Your hormones can't run on empty and neither can you.

Addressing the Root Cause

I have always been intrigued by our hormonal system since every action we take affects it, and I researched extensively in order to learn how it operates. I became a Hormone Cure Coach, so I could teach Dr. Sara Gottfried's Hormone Cure Protocol and help woman get to the root cause and resolve hormonal imbalances. Learn more about this program at https://nourishingsoulutions.com/work-with-me/navigating-hormone-harmony/

The unwillingness of mainstream medicine to delve into the root cause of hormonal imbalance never ceases to amaze me. My summer reads included two extremely cutting edge books stressing how essential iodine is for not only your hormone system but every cell in your body. This is something you won't learn about at your annual physical. But that's another book.

"After 20 years of practicing medicine, I can say it's impossible to achieve your optimal health if you do not have adequate iodine levels. I have yet to see any item that is more important to promoting health or optimizing the function of the immune system than iodine."

– David Brownstein, M.D.

Creating Hormone Harmony

In so many ways, navigating hormone harmony is essential for women in order to flourish. Our hormones impact our health, especially during the omnipresent fluctuations of perimenopause, menopause, and post menopause. Thankfully, many symptoms can be addressed through simple lifestyle adjustments. Daily choices make a huge impact, and focusing on healthy choices will serve your hormone system well. Stress and an unhealthy diet can wreak havoc on your hormones. In fact, there's both an emotional and physical component to hormone health, so when life is flowing harmoniously in the right direction, there are less triggers to compromise your hormone system. When you restore harmony, you'll find yourself dancing through your life with ease, joy, and vibrancy.

Avoid making choices based solely on the belief that they are good for you for this will obstruct harmony. Take fitness, for instance. It's an important aspect of your well-being, but if you push too hard when you are not feeling well or are fatigued, you will not reap the benefits. Even though my lifestyle includes daily exercise, the best thing I do is listen to my body and rest and take a break when I need one. If you never miss a day of rigorous exercise, consider lightening up when your body needs replenishment. It's so much healthier to make nourishing choices that feel and taste good. There is no need to deprive yourself to thrive.

The Clean Food Connection

When I cleaned up my diet and focused on nutrient dense whole grains, greens, and legumes, I discovered that my PMS symptoms decreased. Who wouldn't want that? I've been coaching women for years about the benefits of whole food cleanses and many of them find that it enhances their mood, promotes overall well-being, and decreases inflammation, hot flashes, and perimenopausal symptoms.

Flourish Focus

"A Woman in harmony with her spirit is like a river flowing. She goes where she will without pretense and arrives at her destination prepared to be herself and only herself. "

— Maya Angelou

Self-Reflection:

Assess your level of well-being in these seven keys areas. Rate them from 1–7.

____ Family

____ Friendship

____ Wellness: health, nutrition, fitness, stress, and sleep

____ Intimacy

____ Spirituality/Faith/Connection

____ Purpose: career, hobbies, volunteer activities

____ Finances

What type of discord is blocking your flow? For low rated areas, list the challenges you are facing.

_____

_____

_____

_____

_____

Write down any ideas you have that will help you to weave more harmony into these areas of your life.

_____

_____

_____

_____

_____

What is making you feel so aligned in the higher rated ones?

_____

_____

_____

_____

_____

Action Steps:

1. Relieving stress is essential to get your life flowing in the right direction. Weaving in harmony requires some quiet time to connect to your essence. Take a few minutes in the morning or night, put your hands on your belly, and inhale and exhale really deeply. Feel your belly fill up on the inhalation and deflate on the exhalation. Notice what you feel and consider jotting your thoughts down on a daily basis.

2. Take notice of how the food and beverages you consume impact your hormonal system. Drinking alcohol and eating processed foods and sugary snacks can exacerbate your system.

3. It's also important to note how your sleep and stress levels affect your hormones. Recently, a client shared with me that when she is more stressed she experiences more hot flashes.

_____

_____

_____

_____

Recipe: Cacao Blast-Energizer Smoothie

Restore energy with a Hormone Healthy Cacao Blast.

Serves 2

Ingredients:

- ¼ cup raw cacao powder (if you love chocolate, you can add more)
- 1 Tbsp maca powder
- 1 Tbsp chia seeds
- 2 dried Medjool dates (you can also use figs or 1-2 Tbsp raw honey)
- 1 avocado
- 6 frozen strawberries (you can also use ½ cup raspberries)
- 2 cups of coconut water (water or almond water are also fine)

Directions:

Blend all ingredients at high speed.

See more at https://www.nourishingsoulutions.com/cacao-blast-energizer-smoothie/

Guiding Words from Flourish Contributor, Margaretha Leverage

While visiting my favorite florist a few months ago, I was delighted to meet this most inspiring woman. I first heard her effervescent voice as she responded to the florist's greeting. She has been a regular customer since the shop opened. No surprise that she is their favorite customer as they said she always brings them sunshine.

—

When asked how she was doing, she said, "Good...I have to be good. I am going to be celebrating my 90th birthday." When I turned around to take in this cheerful and energetic voice, I was in awe of this beautifully vibrant woman with twinkling, sterling blue eyes, perfectly pink lips, an inviting smile, and lovely hairstyle.

I was uncharacteristically drawn to her and knew she had something special to share, so I immediately introduced myself, and we enjoyed a lovely conversation. She imparted so many heartfelt words of wisdom that I wish I had been recording our conversation.

She was profoundly engaging and shared that she had three children, 11 great grandchildren, and lost her husband 28 years earlier. She felt blessed and remarked upon the wonderful life she enjoyed with the man of her dreams. Her eyes lit up when she described her husband, "He was quite a man." After all these years, you could just feel the love.

With her beautiful posture and strength, you would never know that she had broken her pelvis and spent three months in a rehab facility recovering. Most

89-year-old women would have thrown in the towel and remained at the nursing home indefinitely, but not Margaretha. Nothing could keep her down for long. As she stood before me in all her splendor, she was a vision of ageless vibrancy.

Her strength and zest for living was palpable, and her life lessons told of a woman in harmony with her spirit. This was a resilient woman who celebrated and cherished her life, friends, and family, and firmly believed that life was good. Most importantly, she was so grateful for the gifts life has and continues to bestow upon her.

She said, "You can't let anything get you down because you never know what's coming next."

Although she looked and acted so bubbly, she sadly shared that her daughter has cancer. She got a little teary, and even though this was worrisome, she wasn't about to dwell on it. After all, she is a 40 year breast cancer survivor. When I asked her if she attributed her impressive longevity to any significant lifestyle choice, she replied, "No, I just don't believe God thought it was my time. He had other plans for me." Clearly, her deep faith and positive outlook continue to keep her thriving and serving others.

As a well nourished woman of 89, she just recently retired from a 40 year volunteer position at a local hospital. You could tell that supporting others was a way of life for her, and that she learned early on how good it feels to give.

Margaretha is a delightful woman who gives as much as she gets. It seems her secret to flourishing is faith, family, friends, and, of course, service.

CHAPTER 9

Glowing with Inner Beauty

"Nothing makes a woman more beautiful than the belief that she is beautiful."

— Sophia Loren

If we succumb to the entertainment industry's point of view, we can easily overlook the importance of real beauty since we are bombarded with an unhealthy emphasis on external beauty. It's sad because this causes many actresses and women to chase a fleeting fountain of youth. Realistically, we can feel forever young, but we can't look forever young. But by making nourishing choices and prioritizing wellness, we can defy age, nurture our inner beauty, and embrace ageless vibrancy. Vibrant women make the choices that help them flourish with vitality and glow with real beauty. Mindful choices that nurture our essence offer us contentment, peace, vibrancy, love, happiness, and ease.

Cosmetics, a beautiful wardrobe, and plastic surgery cannot surpass what nourishing yourself with healthy foods, rest, exercise, joy, love, laughter, gratitude, happiness, friendship, and serenity can do. It's key to nourish yourself from the inside out. This is what really makes beauty blossom. Pure nourishment like this is priceless, and all it takes is an investment in you.

Investing in Yourself

This investment will offer you multiple benefits. Vibrant women carve out healthy lifestyles that increase vitality, ambition, and a zest for living. They live on purpose, follow their hearts, and flourish. They know how to love and be loved.

"To be beautiful means to be yourself. You don't need to be accepted by others. You need to accept yourself."

—Thich Nhat Hanh

Real Beauty Comes with Real Benefits

So many women approaching the next season talk about investing in surgery to enhance their looks, and I always remind them that the best enhancements come from within. Sleep can do wonders for puffy eyes and dark circles. Laughter releases tension in the face and body, and the increased blood flow brings nutrients to the skin that help us glow. Laughter truly is a beauty elixir, so play funny movies, read funny stories, engage with fun people and activities, or take a laughter yoga class to immerse yourself. You just can't beat the positive effects.

> *"There is nothing more rare, nor more beautiful, than a woman being unapologetically herself; comfortable in her perfect imperfection. To me, that is the true essence of beauty."*
>
> — Steve Maraboli

Engaging in activities you enjoy infuses your body with endorphins that bring out the younger you. Relieving stress with yoga and meditation promotes a flexible mind and body and enhances your complexion. And you can't beat a vivacious sex life with its beauty boost and energizing glow. It makes you feel forever young.

Real beauty is when a woman is comfortable in her own skin, can speak from the heart, and shows up as herself. She looks you in the eye, smiles, and is ready to connect with you. Beauty can be described in numerous ways since it is subject to our point of view.

Beauty Bandits and Beauty Benefits

Beauty benefits are also found in the foods you eat but watch out for beauty bandits that threaten your vitality and are lurking in most processed foods, which contain a plethora of high fructose corn syrup, artificial sweeteners, additives, flavorings, preservatives, and synthetic and genetically modified ingredients.

If vibrancy is your goal, it's important to note the impact of alcohol, sugar, and processed food on your overall health. Not only does indulging in these bring down your mood, but they stand in the way of a healthy glow, deplete your energy, and can easily derail your health. Our bodies just can't metabolize these things like they could in our 20s. I can most certainly vouch for this. So have fun indulging a wee bit, but if you want to flourish, it's vital to focus on real foods with the nutritional value to help you look and feel radiant.

Flourish with Nutrient Dense Flavorful Foods

It's essential to cultivate a lifestyle that focuses on food grown on a farm rather than at a factory. Too much of our food supply has been stripped of its natural taste, nutrients, and inherent qualities. Choose foods closest to their natural form that don't require a label. For example, women flourish on a diet filled with fresh fruit, cruciferous vegetables and greens, legumes, nuts, whole and sprouted grains, high quality organic plant-based protein, super foods, and healthy fats with moderate portions of animal protein from sustainably raised animals and wild caught fish.

Whole foods taste better, are more nutritious, and satiate you, so don't fall for the hype promoted by the diet foods industry. Even so called "healthy and natural" foods can have a long list of unwanted ingredients. You might be surprised to learn that eating the whole egg is much healthier than just consuming the egg white. Of course, it tastes better, too, but the choline in the yolk actually helps metabolize the protein in the egg white.

Choose Raw Foods for Radiance

A diet high in raw foods – either uncooked or heated at a low temperature or in a dehydrator – during the warmer months is ideal for radiance. Raw foods are especially nutritious since they are delivered to your system with the enzymes intact, whereas cooked food depletes many of the naturally occurring enzymes. Incorporating raw foods into your daily diet will most certainly help you glow with gorgeousness. Choosing salad, fruit and vegetable snacks, smoothies and freshly squeezed juice are ideal ways to increase your consumption, revitalize, and reduce cravings.

Just think about how flourishing foods make you feel. Typically they boost or restore energy, put you in a better mood, relieve stress, and increase clarity. They can increase libido, satiate you, decrease cravings, help you thrive, and when eaten consistently promote hormone harmony and longevity. Simply put, flourishing foods keep everything flowing, decrease perimenopausal and menopausal symptoms, and help you feel fit, fine, and fabulous.

Make Food an Adventure

Ideally, you want to maintain flexibility in your diet and be open to trying healthy delights. There is no one diet that suits everyone since we are all unique. So, carve out the eating lifestyle that suits you best.

Fat Is Your Friend

Too many women get caught up in no fat or low fat diets and fear fat when healthy fats are absolutely vital for their well-being. When we strip food of essential fats, we lose out on important nutrients. Do you know that your brain is made up of 60 percent fat? Therefore, it responds very poorly to lowfat diets. You need to feed your brain with high quality fats, so that your brain can create the healthiest cells possible. So, go ahead and savor those healthy fats you've been avoiding.

Water

And don't ever underestimate the importance of water since your body thrives on it just like a blossoming flower. Water works wonders for your complexion and your well-being. It's essential to drink an abundance of water, avoid processed foods, and choose organic, non GMO and local foods that satiate you and make you feel good.

Flourishing Foods for Beauty

- Coconuts, coconut oil, and coconut flakes
- Avocados, eggs from pastured hens, olives, olive oil, flax seed oil, and walnut oil
- Wild caught salmon, sardines, high quality fish oils, and oysters
- Super foods like cacao, maca, chia and flax seeds, raw honey, and goji berries
- Greens like kale, Swiss chard, watercress, dandelion, beet greens, and spinach
- Hydrating fruits and vegetables like cucumbers, celery, and watermelon

- Nuts: walnuts, cashews, almonds, Brazil nuts, macadamia nuts, and pumpkin seeds
- Berries: strawberries, blueberries, raspberries, blackberries, etc.
- Antioxidant rich fruits and vegetables like carrots, tomatoes, radishes, and garlic
- Quinoa, millet, and buckwheat
- Legumes: garbanzo beans, peas, black beans, lentils, etc.
- Sea vegetables: nori, arame, dulse, kombu, etc.
- Fermented foods: kombucha, kimchi, fermented soy-tempeh, tamari, and miso

Flourish Focus

"The beauty of a woman is not in the clothes she wears, the figure that she carries, or the way she combs her hair. The beauty of a woman is seen in her eyes, because that is the doorway to her heart, the place where love resides. True beauty in a woman is reflected in her soul. It's the caring that she lovingly gives, the passion that she shows and the beauty of a woman only grows with passing years."

– Audrey Hepburn

Self-Reflection:

What makes you feel beautiful?

_____

_____

_____

_____

_____

_____

_____

_____

_____

_____

Action Steps:

1. Look in the mirror and name one thing that makes you feel beautiful.
   Repeat daily if desired.

2. Treat yourself to a daily dose of beauty food.

3. Beauty tip: If you wake up with puffy eyes (allergies, salt, fatigue, hormones), keep a metal spoon in your freezer, and first thing in the morning, press it gently around your orbital area and lightly on the eyelid. Repeat three times. It feels awesome and is an instant eye-opener and depuffer *(courtesy of Carolan Deacon)*.

Recipe: Nourish-up Chocado

Enjoy this raw chocolate mousse for breakfast, lunch, dinner, or dessert.

Makes 4 servings

Ingredients:

- ½ cup coconut water (water is fine)
- 1 cup baby spinach (dandelion or chard work well)
- 1 avocado
- 4–6 frozen strawberries
- 2 Tbsp raw cacao
- 1 Tbsp maca
- 2 Tbsp chia seeds
- 1 tsp Pure Vanilla Extract
- ¼ cup coconut flakes
- pitted soaked dates or raw honey, optional

Directions:

1. Combine all ingredients except coconut flakes in a blender (works great in a Vitamix).
2. Adjust the amount of coconut water slightly to achieve the right texture.
3. Top with coconut flakes

See more at https://www.nourishingsoulutions.com/nourish-up-chocado

Guiding Words from Flourish Contributor, Mary Costanza

I have been nourished by Mary Costanza's beautiful words for years. She is a gifted writer that shines her light on women.

—

What has my over 40 face seen? It's seen the truth and the realization that with each passing year we become more beautiful. I believe our physical features become strongly defined; it's who we are and what we have been through. But it's not just our physical features. It's our heart and soul that changes as well.

My after 40 face knows what the word 'genuine' truly means. I've had a passion for learning, questioning and disagreeing, and for standing up for what I believe in. I embrace wisdom and my own transformation.

Am I comfortable in my 40s? Absolutely! I proudly wear this face because I have been through a lot, and the woman in the mirror who looks back at me is strong, courageous, and doesn't hate what she sees anymore. She takes care and protects herself.

Would I ever trade my after 40 face for a younger one? Absolutely not because this face has seen too much and now embraces what true beauty is: a strong connection to oneself. This is worth more than any face cream, plastic surgery, or Botox procedure. I don't want to erase or go back in time. I want to keep moving forward, gaining years, wisdom, love, and knowledge. I believe as we age we become classy, sophisticated, and successful beyond measure because we finally know who we are and nothing and nobody can ever take that away from us or turn us into something we don't want to be.

Guiding Words from Flourish Contributor, Tracy Neely

I had the pleasure of connecting with Tracy via the virtual world of health and wellness. As a nutritionist, health and beauty expert, licensed Esthetician, and author, Tracy offers an inspiring message about feeling beautiful and vibrant by embracing your body and focusing on healthy living.

—

As a Women's Health Coach, you may be surprised to know that I didn't always love to exercise. I wanted to enhance my body image, but I wasn't a fan of working out. Although my mother played basketball in high school, ran track, and loved dancing around the house, we didn't discuss the notion of exercising for wellness. Now that I'm a mom, showing my son how important and fun exercise is for our health is vital.

I've always enjoyed being out in nature, so it was easy to go on hikes, rollerblade, or go walking. Long before I made the decision to go back to school to pursue my passion for health and wellness, I had a different perception of exercise. I realize now that I just needed to explore ways to move my body that excited me.

Today, I emphasize the importance of finding enjoyable fitness activities that involve cardio, strength training, and stretching that works for them. I thank God every day for my workout partners and trainer, Natasha. She helped me change the definition of my body, and the workout camaraderie is priceless.

Every day, I make a conscious effort to nourish my body with delicious healthy foods that make me feel good physically and emotionally. I celebrate life by living it to the fullest. The motto I live by is that beauty is a state of mind that connects to the heart and emanates throughout the body.

I hope you feel inspired to take your first step. Learning to embrace my body has been an incredible journey, and I feel such gratitude toward the women all over the world that are taking a stand to live their lives vibrantly.

CHAPTER 10

Thriving with Passion and Purpose

"To breathe your own truth is your heart's most burning desire. To live your purpose is your soul's lifelong dream."

— Dodinsky

A huge part of stepping into a season of ageless vibrancy is discovering your passion and purpose. What gets your juices flowing and helps you thrive? Perhaps you have already found your passion and purpose. Even so, you may be ready for something new. One of the best things about maturing is that you have the opportunity to learn from your mistakes.

By now you've likely recognized that everyone has flaws, challenges, strengths, and weaknesses. No one has it all figured out. Learning this really encourages women to let go of perfection, get off the treadmill of life, and relax into themselves. I am certain that you've developed the courage to stand up for yourself and what you believe without worrying what others will think. After all the years of trying to measure up, isn't it refreshing and empowering to show up as you?

As you usher in the next season, you have the opportunity to address the desires you may have tucked away. Women devote the majority of their lives to doing things for others, but now is your time to ease into you.

"Ten thousand flowers in spring, the moon in autumn, a cool breeze in summer, snow in winter. If your mind isn't clouded by unnecessary things, this is the best season of your life."

— Wu-men (1183-1260), Chinese poet

Now Is the Time for You

This is your chance to write a new chapter. Plant the flowers you always wanted in your garden and infuse your life with color. You have the option to carve out a path of fulfillment in this pivotal stage of your life in whatever form you choose. Now is the time to access your dreams and desires.

"The recipe to a fulfilling life is simple and gratifying: reconnect with the light within, unmute your soul, and restore its voice"

— Liliana C. Vanasco

Back in my early 30s, I read a book titled Women's Bodies Women's Wisdom, which I mentioned earlier. The author stressed how women, especially mothers, need to reclaim their essence to find their passion and purpose in their next season. As mothers, we easily lose ourselves in childrearing and can feel a bit lost when our children leave the nest. The author explained how our well-being can become compromised when we feel stuck or unfulfilled.

My Mom, My Role Model

My resilient mom modeled a passion for living, learning, and pursuing her dreams. As a young mother of three little children, she went back to school to be a teacher, which was absolutely her passion. This fulfilling career helped her thrive both personally, socially, and financially. Although she worked very hard, this afforded her a lovely life-style. After my Dad died, she even married a fellow colleague that she had cultivated a close friendship with. She is now retired and enjoys her family, traveling around the world with her husband, learning something new every day, and best of all, she and her husband are infused with joy, love, and laughter.

Spread Your Wings, Broaden Your Horizon

Like many women, I cherished my role as a stay at home mom and found nurturing my four kids and being of service in the community very fulfilling, but I always knew that I would birth a new idea, project, or business in my life. As a busy mom of two daughters with two sons yet to be born, I wasn't quite ready to focus on that yet, so I tucked those thoughts away.

I am grateful that this seed was planted back then because one of the best decisions I ever made was to get certified to be a health coach in my 40s. It felt like giving birth to a new part of me that offered a sense of passion and purpose. I felt so exhilarated that I nicknamed my pursuit Baby 5. Now at 50, as my kids grow older and leave the nest, I continue to blossom with a fulfilling career.

I've seen many women stagnate after their children leave the nest, so it's vitally important to begin addressing your desires before they leave the nest, too. I am so proud when I see friends and clients reinvent themselves. A few years back, a client and special friend landed a position as a director of a nursery school. Recently, a client shared her plans with me to get a degree in social work. Life is a long time even though it flies by, so why not use your unique talents to pursue an avenue that really speaks to you?

Up until now, you may have devoted your life to child rearing, community service, caring for loved ones, a fulfilling career, or a job that paid the bills, but now it's up to you to decide to continue with what you've been doing, retire, or change course. The sky is the limit, so dig deep and listen.

"Our dreams and aspirations are the gateways to our deepest joy. Follow those dreams and watch your life flourish!"

— Mary Byrne, Garden of Pensiveness

Presently, your life may not afford you the opportunity for change, and this is fine, but you can still consider how you want to live out the next season. Explore your answers to the questions below and start planning and preparing for living a life with passion and purpose.

Flourish Focus

"It is confidence in our bodies, minds, and spirits that allow us to keep looking for new adventures, new directions to grow in, and new lessons to learn – which is what life is all about."

— Oprah Winfrey

Self-Reflection:

What do you dream about doing?

_____

_____

_____

_____

What are you passionate about?

_____

_____

_____

_____

What lights you up inside?

_____

_____

_____

Is there an organization in your community that could use your time and talents?

_____

_____

_____

_____

Have you already found your purpose, or does it need more time to emerge? If you have found your purpose, please describe it.

_____

_____

_____

_____

What is your heart's fancy?

_____

_____

_____

_____

Action Step:

Take a chance and try something new that interests you (i.e. taking a class, developing a new hobby or activity, or participating in community service).

List some ideas:

_____

_____

_____

_____

Recipe: Raw Dark Chocolate Sauce

Enjoy a truly delectable indulgence.

Ingredients:

- 1 cup raw cacao powder
- 1 cup raw honey
- 1 cup almond butter

Directions:

1. Mix all ingredients together in a blender or food processor.
2. Serve with fruit for dipping.

See more at https://www.nourishingsoulutions.com/raw-dark-chocolate-sauce/

Guiding Words from Flourish Contributor, Marie Magnani

I had the pleasure of meeting the loving, charming, vibrant, and soulful Marie, aka Aunt Marie, through her niece, Lorri, who shared her aunt's zest for living, when I told her about the book I was writing. I really appreciated Marie's friendly, lovely, and forthcoming demeanor filled with laughter and smiles.

—

Aunt Marie was born in Italy, immigrated to the USA, and just celebrated her 99th birthday. She lived a good life with her five brothers in the Bronx as Nonie's right hand (her mom). She never felt deprived or poor in this simpler time; she admired her resilient mother for raising her family primarily as a single parent. Nonie lived to be 100 years old (and nine months) and inspired a love of cooking in Marie.

Marie had an affinity for learning and loved school. Even though the polio she suffered as a little girl caused her left side to be lower than the right, she never used that as a crutch. She never missed a day of school even when her mom was hospitalized. Rather than miss a single day, she brought her 4-year-old brother, Rudy, with her. She was still tickled by "Little Rudy," now 87, and was so happy that he moved in after his wife passed.

It's no surprise that Marie became a stellar teacher dedicated to her students and colleagues. Her favorite grade was 6th, and she still keeps up with some of her 6th grade students. She was extremely nurturing and a devoted mentor to her fellow teachers and principals.

Although Marie didn't have much opportunity for dating, she enjoyed a large circle of friends and family and an adventurous life. She described a beautiful trip to her birthplace in Italy and recalled a fabulous 6-week tour in Europe where she country hopped by ship and enjoyed traveling around the U.S.A.

While teaching was her passion and gift to the world, family life always fed Marie's soul. She's so grateful for living a rich life with her nurturing family. She was blessed with many loving nieces, nephews, grand nieces and nephews, and took them on an array of adventures. Everyone loved being with Aunt Marie. In fact, some of them even came to live with her. Although she explains with a little surprise that most of her college friends are gone, she happily enjoys socializing with her church friends.

She still lives in the home her family moved to on Long Island in 1950. After retiring from an impressive teaching career at 68 to take care of her ailing mom, Marie began volunteering at Good Samaritan Hospital. Volunteering was a great fit, and she just retired last year due to her arthritic hands and hindered stability. Not quite ready to throw in the towel, she is now helping to record this hospital's history for its guild. Imagine volunteering for 50 years?

When I asked what she attributes her long vibrant life to, she beautifully said, The Blessed Mother has always held my hand through the toughest moments of my life. ng I don't think I will ever forget the way she shared these words. As we chatted, she caressed her rosary beads just like my Nana used to do. She described how prayer opens your heart and mind and has always been a constant in her life.

Marie's Nourishing Nuggets

- *"God is good."*
- *"Don't waste time being mad or angry."*
- *"You need to know when to shut up because you're not going to change someone's mind."*
- *"Don't rush through life; it goes fast enough as it is."*
- *"Life is too short no matter how long it is."* Somehow, I didn't expect a 99–year-old woman to say this.

Guiding Words from Flourish Contributor, Nancy Mindes

I had the pleasure of meeting Nancy about 10 years ago at Divine Yoga (now RVC Yoga). At 60–something, Nancy has lived an interesting journey and sets the tone for reinventing your career to suit your lifestyle.

—

"Trust your intuition; it's just like going fishin'."

— Paul Simon

Before I took a deep dive into psychoanalysis, the human potential movement, training with 7 Habits founder, Stephen Covey, Landmark Education, Coach U, Enlightened Warrior and Wizard Training camps, being a yogi, Pilates practitioner, trance dancer, and meditator, I was a human doing. I was an ambitious-to-be-somebody 38-year-old.

It was my belief that it was important to be a superstar in every area of life. What I discovered on my journey was that an ego-based rather than heart-centered desire was costing me big time. What I was getting was not what I wanted.

Every few months after being on the merry go-round to what seemed like success, the big collapse would take place on the couch with bronchitis and general exhaustion. Those were the moments I started to think, "Hmm. Something is not quite right." I had to ask myself, "Whose ideal life am I really trying to live?"

I knew that for peace of mind I would be well served to listen to the whispers of my intuition and find another definition of success. I listened to my heart and reinvented my career to suit my lifestyle by completing 3+ years of professional coach training. When I turned 50, my transformation led to opportunities to guide women toward reinventing their lives.

"Why are you knocking on every other door? Go knock at the door of your own heart."

– Rumi

Each of us has our own idea of how to define flourish. To me it means to thrive and grow luxuriantly.

Here are a few things I had to learn (and re-learn) along the way:

- *Do work you love, and the universe will pull you along.*
- *Don't compare yourself to others.*
- *Draw. Write. Paint. Garden.*
- *Eat only foods that nourish you (break up with Pop-Tarts).*
- *Give up blame and complaints when you talk. (You may find you have very little to say.)*

- *Hug.*
- *Invest in a fulfilling life.*
- *Let go of time suckers and dump emotional vampires.*
- *Live as if there is only this moment. (Yup, that's it!)*
- *Practice yoga. Stretch yourself. Lighten up. Meditate.*
- *Shake your booty. Laugh. Dance. Skate. Sing (even if it is only in the shower).*
- *Uncover what feeds your soul and go do it.*
- *Watch what you say to yourself. (Treat yourself like a dear friend.)*

What does your heart tell you? Make your own list. Begin. The rest is easy.

There's a Present Just Waiting to be Unwrapped

Now that you've read the book and embraced a path of vibrant living, I hope this has given you the space to connect with your essence and consider your choices, your journey, your gifts, your dreams, goals, and desires.

I hope it's inspired you to fall in love with you, your life, and all that you have to look forward to. It's about time you start celebrating and nourishing you! Now that you've embraced your sensuality, wisdom, and grace, I hope you are excited to embrace the opportunities and adventures this season can offer you.

By nurturing your garden and filling your fountain of youth, you'll design each decade mindfully, discover your sweet spot, weave in a sense of harmony, radiate beauty, and thrive with renewed passion and purpose. So go ahead and reclaim your zest for living and blossom with a bountiful life full of fun, joy, pleasure, love, and fulfillment. May you always feel forever young, and may these meaningful words motivate you to open up the beautiful gift waiting for you — your future!

"In terms of days and moments lived, you'll never again be as young as you are right now, so spend this day, the youth of your future, in a way that deflects regret. Invest in yourself. Have some fun. Do something important. Love somebody extra."

— Victoria Moran

Now that you have embraced a zest for life, may you always feel forever vibrant and flourish.

FLOURISH READING LIST

Bhajan. *The Aquarian Teacher.* Fourth edition. KRI. 2007.

Brownstein, David. *Iodine: Why You Need It, Why You Can't Live Without It.* 2009.

Byrne, Mary. *The Garden Of Pensiveness.* https://www.facebook.com/pages/The-Garden-Of-Pensiveness/367268523352486

Chapman, Gary D. *The 5 Love Languages: The Secret to Love That Lasts.* 2010.

Chopra, Deepak. *Ageless Body, Timeless Mind: The Quantum Alternative to Growing Old.* 1994.

David, Marc. *Mind/Body Nutrition - Increase your energy, eat without stress, and transform your health.* 2006.

Estés, Clarissa Pinkola. *Women Who Run with the Wolves.* 1996.

Farrow, Lynne and David Brownstein M.D. *The Iodine Crisis: What You Don't Know About Iodine Can Wreck Your Life.* 2013.

Gottfried, Sara, M.D. *The Hormone Cure: Reclaim Balance, Sleep and Sex Drive; Lose Weight; Feel Focused, Vital, and Energized Naturally with the Gottfried Protocol.* 2013.

Hempel, Amy. *The Collected Stories of Amy Hempel.* 2007.

Hyman, Mark. *The Blood Sugar Solution: The Ultra-Healthy Program for Losing Weight, Preventing Disease, and Feeling Great Now.* 2012.

Khalsa, Gurmukh Kaur and Cathryn Michon. *The Eight Human Talents: Restore the Balance and Serenity within You with Kundalini Yoga.* 2001.

Laughter Yoga. http://laughteryoga.org/english/home

"Meditation for a Calm Heart." Kundalini Yoga as Taught By Yogi Bhajan. http://www.yogibhajan.org/ybkriyas/index.php?id=87

Metz, Pamela K., Tobin, Jaequeline. *The Tao of Women.* 1995.

Moran, Victoria. *Creating a Charmed Life: Sensible, Spiritual Secrets Every Busy Woman Should Know.* 1999.

Northrup, Christiane, M.D. *Women's Bodies, Women's Wisdom: Creating Physical and Emotional Health and Healing.* Revised Edition. 2010.

— *The Wisdom of Menopause: Creating Physical and Emotional Health During the Change.* Revised Edition. 2012.

Rosenthal, Joshua. *Integrative Nutrition: Feed Your Hunger for Health and Happiness.* 3rd Edition. 2014.

Whitehouse, Maureen. *Soul-Full Eating: A (Delicious) Path to Higher Consciousness.* 2007.

FLOURISH BEYOND 50 CONTRIBUTORS

- Polly Leaf
- Jane Stinson-www.janestinson.com
- Carolan Deacon-www.carolandeacon.com
- Patsie Smith-www.patsiesmith.com
- Liz Murray-www.lizmurraywellness.com
- Jayne Justice-www.jaynejustice.com
- Samyak Yamauchi-www.samyakyamauchi.com
- Margaretha Leverage
- Mary Costanza-www.facebook.com/
  marycostanzaheartandsoul
- Tracy Neely- www.tracyneely.com
- Marie Magnani
- Nancy Mindes-www.fancynancysays.com

Learn more about each one of these vibrant women on my blog at http://nourishingsoulutions.com/blog/

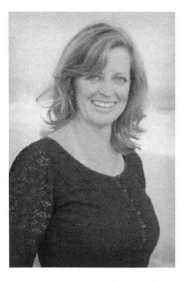

Meet Judy Griffin, CHHC, AADP

As a nutrition and lifestyle coach, workplace wellness educator, retreat presenter, speaker, teacher and writer, Judy shares her expertise, affinity for soulful wellness, and passion for cooking to help women nourish their way to a vibrant life.

After experiencing a tragic loss at the age of 40, Judy chose vibrant nourishment as a recovery tool. With a reclaimed zest for life she began to flourish and is determined to inspire other women to feel fit, fabulous, and flourish at any age. Judy believes that embracing pleasure, play, and joy is essential in reclaiming youthful vitality.

Judy is a graduate of Institute for Integrative Nutrition, is Level 1 Raw Food Certified, a Level 1 Reiki Practitioner, a Certified Hormone Cure Coach, the owner of Nourishing Soulutions and a Founding Partner at Vital Advantage Consulting.

Judy received a B.S. from SUNY Oneonta and worked in investment management for 7 years until she switched hats to raise her four children. She resides in Rockville Centre, N.Y. with her husband and two teenaged sons. One daughter attends college, while the other daughter has already left the nest.

As a multi-passionate wellness enthusiast, Judy loves to cook up healthy delights and explore the many ways to have fun with fitness. You'll often find her hopping around the neighborhood in her Kangoo Jumps, swim-ming in the ocean, bike riding or practicing yoga. She squeezes the most out of each day, celebrates each sunset, and often stays up way too late.

Judy has a gift for teaching women how to nourish to flourish and believes that when women thrive so do their loved ones. One client described her as *"a special woman who truly cares about our health, and in doing such, she educates us with love,"* while another said, *"she is a wealth of knowledge and a pleasure to work with. It is NOT about being thin. It is about getting through this thing we call "LIFE." Healthy in mind, body, and spirit. That is what Judy offers."*

photo courtesy of bsquaredphotography.net

Are you ready to embrace vibrant living and flourish?

Invite Judy Griffin, to speak at your workplace, club, civic association, women's group, community center, health club, wellness center, yoga studio, college, school, library, professional organization, or any other venue.

Judy offers one on one coaching, Hormone Harmony group series, guided cleanses, Diabetes Wellness Classes, cooking classes, and workplace wellness. Judy writes a weekly newsletter and blog and also writes for a few online magazines. *Flourish Beyond 50* is her first book.

Her mission of this book is to convey to women that this is just the beginning and they have the power to design a fulfilling, joyful, and vivacious life. This is a time for women to nurture their garden so they can fully blossom.

Come join the conversation at www.facebook.com/Flourishbeyond50.

Look out for Flourish Beyond 50 Retreats and connect with Judy to learn about upcoming programs, classes and how you can work with her at:

www.Flourishbeyond50.com
judy@flourishbeyond50.com
www.facebook.com/NourishingSoulutions
www.vitaladvantageconsulting.com